BASIC
ETHICS

EXAMINING ETHICS
IN A HEALTHCARE SETTING

R. L. COHEN, PHD

Humanities
ACADEMIC PUBLISHERS

ISBN: 9781988557526 (Paperback)
ISBN: 9781988557540 (Hardcover)

Published: 2024

Published in the United States of America
Published by Humanities Academic Publishers

TABLE OF CONTENTS

CHAPTER 1

DEFINE ETHICS IN HEALTHCARE

The study of ethics in healthcare involves a comprehensive examination of the moral principles, values, and responsibilities that guide healthcare professionals in their practice and decision-making processes. This field encompasses various aspects, including normative ethics, moral character, ethical decision-making, and professional responsibilities within healthcare settings. In healthcare, normative ethics focuses on identifying and justifying the moral norms that should govern healthcare professionals' behavior. It involves determining ethical principles and guidelines that guide ethical conduct in healthcare practice. Normative ethics in healthcare plays a crucial role in guiding the behavior of healthcare professionals by establishing moral norms and ethical principles that govern their actions.

One of the key ethical principles in healthcare is beneficence, which emphasizes the obligation of healthcare providers to act in the best interest of their patients and to promote their well-being. This principle underscores the importance of healthcare professionals making decisions that benefit their patients and prioritize their health outcomes. Another fundamental ethical principle in healthcare is nonmaleficence, which requires healthcare professionals to do no harm to their patients.

This principle highlights the importance of avoiding actions that may cause harm or worsen the condition of patients. Healthcare providers are ethically obligated to prioritize the safety and well-being of their patients, as well as minimize any potential risks associated with their care.

Autonomy is another essential ethical principle in healthcare that emphasizes the right of patients to make informed decisions about their own care. Healthcare professionals are required to respect the autonomy of their patients by providing them with relevant information, involving them in decision-making processes, and respecting their choices regarding treatment options. Respecting patient autonomy is crucial to upholding the dignity and rights of individuals seeking healthcare services.

Justice is also a significant ethical principle in healthcare that pertains to the fair and equitable distribution of healthcare resources and services. Healthcare professionals are ethically obligated to ensure that healthcare resources are allocated fairly, without discrimination or bias, and that all patients have equal access to quality care. Upholding principles of justice in healthcare practice helps to promote fairness, equality, and social responsibility within the healthcare system. Normative ethics in healthcare plays a vital role in guiding healthcare professionals' behavior by establishing ethical principles and moral norms that govern their actions.

Beneficence, nonmaleficence, autonomy, and justice are key ethical principles that guide ethical conduct in healthcare practice and help to ensure the delivery of high-quality, patient-centered care. By adhering to these ethical principles, healthcare professionals can uphold the values of compassion, integrity, and respect in their interactions with patients and contribute to the promotion of ethical healthcare practices.

Normative Ethics

In healthcare, normative ethics focuses on identifying and justifying the moral norms that should govern healthcare professionals' behavior. It involves determining ethical principles and guidelines that guide ethical conduct in healthcare practice. Normative ethics in healthcare plays a critical role in guiding healthcare professionals' behavior by establishing moral norms and ethical principles that govern their actions. One of the key ethical principles in healthcare is beneficence, which emphasizes the obligation of healthcare providers to act in the best interest of their patients and to promote their well-being. This principle underscores the importance of healthcare professionals making decisions that benefit their patients and prioritize their health outcomes.

Another fundamental ethical principle in healthcare is nonmaleficence, which requires healthcare professionals to do no harm to their patients. This principle highlights the importance of avoiding actions that may cause harm or worsen the condition of patients. Healthcare providers are ethically obligated to prioritize the safety and well-being of their patients, as well as minimize any potential risks associated with their care. Autonomy is another essential ethical principle in healthcare that emphasizes the right of patients to make informed decisions about their own care. Healthcare professionals are required to respect their patients' autonomy by providing them with relevant information, involving them in decision-making processes, and respecting their treatment options. Respecting patient autonomy is crucial to upholding the dignity and rights of individuals seeking healthcare services. Justice is also a significant ethical principle in healthcare that pertains to the fair and equitable distribution of healthcare resources and services. Healthcare professionals are ethically obligated to ensure that healthcare resources are allocated fairly, without discrimination or bias, and that all patients have equal access to quality care. Upholding principles of justice in healthcare practice helps to promote fairness, equality, and social responsibility within the healthcare system. Normative ethics in healthcare plays a vital role in guiding the behavior of healthcare professionals by establishing ethical principles and moral norms that govern their actions. Beneficence, nonmaleficence, autonomy, and justice are key ethical principles that guide ethical conduct in healthcare practice and help to ensure the delivery of high-quality, patient-centered care. By adhering to these ethical principles, healthcare professionals can uphold the values of compassion, integrity, and respect in their interactions with patients and contribute to the promotion of ethical healthcare practices.

Moral Character and Virtue Ethics

The study of moral character and virtue ethics emphasizes the importance of cultivating virtuous traits such as compassion, integrity, and empathy in healthcare professionals to uphold ethical standards and provide compassionate care to patients. The study of moral character and virtue ethics in healthcare underscores the significance of cultivating virtuous traits such as compassion, integrity, and empathy among healthcare professionals to uphold ethical standards and deliver compassionate care to patients. Virtue ethics, as a normative ethical theory, focuses on the moral character of individuals and emphasizes the development of virtuous traits that guide ethical decision-making and behavior. In healthcare, cultivating virtues such as compassion is essential for healthcare professionals to demonstrate empathy and understanding towards patients, thereby fostering trust and promoting patient well-being. Compassion enables healthcare providers to connect with patients on a deeper level, acknowledge their suffering, and provide care with kindness and empathy. Integrity is another crucial virtue in healthcare that involves honesty, transparency, and adherence to ethical principles. Healthcare professionals with integrity demonstrate a commitment to truthfulness, ethical conduct, and accountability in their interactions with patients, colleagues, and the broader healthcare system. Upholding integrity helps to build trust, maintain professional credibility, and ensure the ethical practice of healthcare. Empathy is a fundamental virtue in healthcare that involves the ability to understand and share the feelings of patients, demonstrating care, concern, and emotional support. Healthcare professionals who cultivate empathy can establish meaningful relationships with patients, address their emotional needs, and provide holistic care that considers their physical, emotional, and psychological well-being.

Ethical Decision-Making

Ethics in healthcare also involves exploring ethical decision-making processes and addressing ethical dilemmas that healthcare professionals may encounter in their practice. This includes navigating conflicting moral norms, balancing ethical considerations, and making informed and ethically sound decisions in healthcare settings. Professional responsibilities and ethical competence are essential components of the study of ethics in healthcare, focusing on the ability of healthcare professionals to uphold ethical standards, provide patient-centered care, and navigate complex ethical challenges with integrity and moral excellence.

Ethics in healthcare encompasses the exploration of ethical decision-making processes and the resolution of ethical dilemmas that healthcare professionals may face in their practice. This involves navigating conflicting moral norms, balancing ethical considerations, and making informed and ethically sound decisions in healthcare settings. Professional responsibilities and ethical competence are integral components of the study of ethics in healthcare, emphasizing the importance of healthcare professionals upholding ethical standards, delivering patient-centered care, and effectively managing complex ethical challenges with integrity and moral excellence. In the healthcare context, ethical decision-making involves a systematic process of identifying ethical issues, considering relevant ethical principles and guidelines, evaluating alternative courses of action, and making decisions that align with ethical standards and the best interests of patients. Healthcare professionals are often confronted with ethical dilemmas that require careful deliberation, ethical reasoning, and a commitment to upholding moral values and professional responsibilities. Addressing ethical dilemmas in healthcare requires healthcare professionals to navigate conflicting moral norms, such as the principles of beneficence, nonmaleficence, autonomy, and justice, while considering the unique circumstances of each situation and the preferences of patients. Balancing these ethical considerations involves weighing the potential benefits and harms of different courses of action, respecting patient autonomy and rights, promoting fairness and equity in healthcare delivery, and prioritizing the well-being and safety of patients. Professional responsibilities in healthcare encompass a range of ethical obligations, including maintaining patient confidentiality, obtaining informed consent, providing competent and compassionate care, advocating for patient welfare, and collaborating with colleagues to ensure quality healthcare delivery. Ethical competence involves the ability of healthcare professionals to apply ethical principles, guidelines, and decision-making frameworks in practice, engage in ethical reflection and dialogue, and respond effectively to ethical challenges and dilemmas that arise in healthcare settings. Ethics in healthcare involves exploring ethical decision-making processes, addressing ethical dilemmas, navigating conflicting moral norms, balancing ethical considerations, and upholding professional responsibilities and ethical competence. By fostering a strong ethical foundation, healthcare professionals can provide patient-centered care, navigate complex ethical challenges with integrity, and contribute to the promotion of ethical healthcare practices and patients' well-being.

By studying ethics in healthcare, healthcare professionals, policymakers, and researchers gain a deeper understanding of the ethical considerations, moral responsibilities, and values that underpin ethical healthcare practice. This knowledge helps guide ethical decision-making, promote patient-centered care, and uphold ethical standards in healthcare delivery, ultimately contributing to the well-being and rights of patients and the broader community.

Why Study Different Professional Ethics Standards

The study of ethics in healthcare involves a comprehensive examination of the moral principles, values, and responsibilities that guide healthcare professionals in their practice and decision-making processes. This field encompasses various aspects, including normative ethics, moral character, ethical decision-making, and professional responsibilities within healthcare settings. Healthcare professionals are guided by professional codes of ethics specific to their respective fields, such as nursing, psychology, and dentistry. These codes outline the ethical standards, values, and responsibilities that professionals are expected to uphold in their practice. Membership bodies and professional organizations play a crucial role in establishing and promoting ethical guidelines within each profession. For example, in nursing, the American Nurses Association (ANA) and the

International Council of Nurses (ICN) are prominent membership bodies that provide ethical guidance and support for nurses worldwide. In psychology, the American Psychological Association (APA) and the British Psychological Society (BPS) offer ethical guidelines and resources for psychologists. Dentists adhere to ethical standards set by organizations such as the American Dental Association (ADA) and the General Dental Council (GDC) in the UK. By studying different professional codes of healthcare ethics and understanding the ethical guidelines established by membership bodies in each profession, healthcare professionals can enhance their ethical competence, uphold ethical standards, and provide high-quality care to patients. The study of ethics in healthcare is essential for promoting ethical conduct, ensuring patient well-being, and maintaining healthcare practice integrity across various disciplines.

Four Major Principles in Bioethics

James Childress and Thomas Beauchamp are two prominent bioethicists known for their influential work in bioethics. They co-authored the book "Principles of Biomedical Ethics," which has become a foundational text in the field of bioethics. Childress and Beauchamp are recognized for their development of the four--principles approach to bioethics, which includes the principles of respect for autonomy, nonmaleficence, beneficence, and justice. Their work has had a significant impact on ethical decision-making in healthcare, shaping the ethical framework used in medical practice and research.

Respect for Autonomy

This principle underscores the necessity of respecting individuals' rights to make informed healthcare decisions. It involves honoring their preferences, choices, and decisions, ensuring they have the autonomy to make their own treatment choices. Respect for autonomy is a fundamental ethical principle in healthcare that emphasizes the importance of honoring individuals' rights to make informed decisions about their own healthcare. This principle underscores the necessity of respecting patients' preferences, choices, and decisions, ensuring that they have the autonomy to make their own treatment choices. Healthcare professionals are ethically obligated to provide patients with relevant information about their health condition, treatment options, risks, and benefits and to involve them in decision-making processes to respect their autonomy. One possible reference that delves into the concept of respect for autonomy in healthcare is Beauchamp & Childress (2013).

This seminal work outlines the four principles of biomedical ethics, including respect for autonomy, beneficence, nonmaleficence, and justice, and discusses how these principles guide ethical decision-making in healthcare. The authors provide in-depth analysis and case studies to illustrate the application of the principle of respect for autonomy in clinical practice, as well as its significance in upholding patient rights and promoting ethical healthcare delivery.

Nonmaleficence

This principle requires healthcare professionals to refrain from causing harm. It mandates prioritizing patients' well-being and safety in all care aspects. Nonmaleficence is a foundational ethical principle in healthcare that requires healthcare professionals to prioritize the well-being and safety of patients by refraining from causing harm. This principle mandates that healthcare providers must strive to prevent harm and minimize risks to patients in all aspects of care delivery. Upholding the principle of nonmaleficence entails a commitment to ethical practice, patient safety, and the avoidance of actions that may harm or adversely affect patients. Beauchamp & Childress (2013) outline the four principles of biomedical ethics, including nonmaleficence, respect for autonomy, beneficence, and justice, and discuss how nonmaleficence is a guide to ethical decision-making in healthcare. Pellegrino & Thomasma (1988) suggest that the ethical principles of beneficence and nonmaleficence in healthcare, focusing on the moral obligation of healthcare professionals to promote the well-being of patients and prevent harm, are vital. The authors discuss the ethical considerations surrounding nonmaleficence, the complexities of balancing risks and benefits in healthcare decision-making, and the importance of upholding patient safety as a core ethical value.

Beneficence

This principle involves the duty to promote patients' well-being and best interests. Healthcare providers should take actions that benefit patients, improve their health outcomes, and enhance their overall welfare. Beneficence is a core ethical principle in healthcare that entails the duty of healthcare providers to promote patients' well-being and best interests. This principle emphasizes the obligation to take actions that benefit patients, improve their health outcomes, and enhance their overall welfare. Healthcare professionals are ethically mandated to prioritize beneficence by providing care that is in the best interest of patients, promoting their health and well-being, and advocating for interventions that optimize their quality of life. Beauchamp & Childress (2013) further suggest that the principle of beneficence highlights the ethical imperative of promoting patient well-being and advocating for actions that benefit patients in clinical practice. Gillon (1994) also explores the philosophical foundations of medical ethics, including the principle of beneficence, and discusses the moral obligations of healthcare professionals to prioritize the well-being and best interests of patients. The author examines the ethical considerations surrounding beneficence, the complexities of balancing risks and benefits in healthcare decision-making, and the importance of upholding patient welfare as a central ethical value in healthcare practice.

Justice

This principle stresses fairness, equity, and resource distribution in healthcare. It calls for equitable treatment of individuals, ensuring equal healthcare access, and addressing systemic inequalities to advance social justice in healthcare delivery. Justice is a fundamental ethical principle in healthcare that emphasizes fairness, equity, and resource distribution. This principle calls for the equitable treatment of individuals, ensuring equal access to healthcare services, and addressing systemic inequalities to advance social justice in healthcare delivery. Healthcare professionals are ethically obligated to promote justice by advocating for fair allocation of resources, reducing disparities in healthcare access, and addressing social determinants of health to improve health outcomes for all individuals. Justice in healthcare focuses on the ethical principles of fairness, equity, and meeting health needs fairly. The moral imperative of addressing health disparities, promoting equal access to healthcare services, and advocating for policies that advance social justice in healthcare delivery is an important aspect of justice. Similarly, the ethical dimensions of justice in healthcare, emphasizing the importance of patient empowerment, autonomy, and participation in healthcare decision-making, are important.

TERMINOLOGY

1. **Normative Ethics** - The branch of ethics concerned with the criteria of what is morally right and wrong. It includes the formulation of moral rules that have implications for what human actions, institutions, and ways of life should be like.

2. **Beneficence** - An ethical principle that refers to actions that promote the well-being of others. In healthcare, it emphasizes the obligation of healthcare providers to act in the best interest of their patients and to promote their well-being.

3. **Nonmaleficence** - An ethical principle that requires healthcare professionals to refrain from causing harm to patients. This principle underlines the necessity to avoid actions that might harm the patient.

4. **Autonomy** - In healthcare ethics, this principle emphasizes the right of patients to make informed decisions about their own medical care. Healthcare providers must provide all necessary information to patients and respect their decisions regarding their treatment.

5. **Justice** - This principle pertains to the fair and equitable distribution of healthcare resources and services. It involves ensuring that all individuals have equal access to healthcare without discrimination or bias.

6. **Moral Character** - Refers to the virtues or ethical traits that a person embodies that guide their behavior. In healthcare, virtues like compassion, integrity, and empathy are crucial for ethical practice.

7. **Virtue Ethics** - An approach in normative ethical theory that emphasizes the virtues, or moral character, as the basis for ethical behavior, rather than rules (deontology) or consequences (consequentialism).

8. **Ethical Decision-Making** - The process involving the evaluation of different choices by applying ethical principles and moral values, aimed at resolving ethical dilemmas, especially significant in healthcare settings where decisions can have profound effects on patient welfare.

9. **Professional Responsibilities** - Obligations that healthcare professionals have towards their patients and society, including maintaining patient confidentiality, obtaining informed consent, and providing competent care.

10. **Ethical Competence** - The ability of healthcare professionals to apply ethical principles and guidelines in their practice, engage in ethical reflection, and respond to ethical challenges effectively.

11. **Bioethics** - A field of study that deals with the ethical implications of biological and medical procedures and technologies, focusing on patient care and medical research.

DISCUSSION QUESTIONS

1. **Autonomy in Pediatric Care:**

   Scenario: A 14-year-old child diagnosed with a terminal illness wants to refuse a painful treatment that could potentially extend their life. The parents wish to proceed with the treatment. Discuss how healthcare professionals should balance the principle of autonomy with beneficence in this scenario.

2. **Nonmaleficence in Emergency Situations:**

   Scenario: Imagine a scenario where an emergency room doctor must quickly decide between two patients who need immediate life-saving surgery but only one operating room is available. How should the doctor apply the principle of nonmaleficence in deciding who to treat first?

3. **Justice in Resource Allocation:**

   Scenario: A small community hospital receives a limited supply of a life-saving drug. There are more patients in need than doses available. How should the hospital distribute the medication fairly, applying the principle of justice?

4. **Beneficence vs. Nonmaleficence:**

   Scenario: Consider a patient in severe pain that requires a high dose of painkillers, potentially hastening death due to side effects. How should healthcare providers decide between the principle of beneficence (relieving pain) and nonmaleficence (avoiding harm)?

5. **Respecting Autonomy in Mental Health:**

   Scenario: A patient with severe depression refuses treatment, believing nothing will help them. Should healthcare professionals override the patient's decision to respect their autonomy or intervene to provide care? Discuss the ethical considerations involved.

6. **Justice and Healthcare Accessibility:**

   Scenario: In a rural area with limited healthcare facilities, patients have unequal access to specialized care. What responsibilities do healthcare providers have to ensure equitable access to all community members?

7. **Conflicting Principles in Public Health Emergencies:**

   Scenario: During a pandemic, a vaccine becomes available but is in short supply. Should healthcare workers prioritize vaccinations for themselves to maintain healthcare services (beneficence) or distribute it first to the elderly and vulnerable (justice)? Discuss the ethical challenges.

8. **Cultural Beliefs and Autonomy:**

   Scenario: A patient's cultural belief prohibits blood transfusions, but such a procedure is necessary to save their life. How should healthcare providers respect cultural differences while still acting in the patient's best health interest?

9. **Professional Integrity and Conflicts of Interest:**

   Scenario: A doctor discovers that a cheaper alternative medication is just as effective as a more expensive drug they have been prescribing, which they receive incentives to promote. Discuss the ethical implications of the doctor's choice regarding beneficence, nonmaleficence, and justice.

10. **Ethical Considerations in End-of-Life Care:**

    Scenario: An elderly patient with advanced dementia has a Do Not Resuscitate (DNR) order, but the family wishes to revoke it against the patient's earlier wishes when they were of sound mind. How should healthcare providers handle this situation respecting the patient's autonomy and the family's wishes?

CHAPTER 2

ETHICAL THEORIES

B ioethics is a field that encompasses a wide range of ethical considerations and moral issues beyond just sexual behavior. It addresses
topics such as healthcare, medical research, patient rights, genetic testing, organ donation, resource allocation, and emerging technologies in
medicine. Bioethics also explores ethical dilemmas related to codes of
behavior, such as actions towards others and theft. It provides a secular
and inclusive ethical framework that promotes ethical decision-making
based on reason, evidence, and the well-being of individuals and communities. Bioethics is influenced by religious teachings and principles
from Judaism, Christianity, and Islam but also transcends religion by
fostering dialogue and collaboration. Meta-ethics and normative ethics
theories help to clarify the ethical landscape and provide guidance for
ethical decision-making in bioethics. Moral realism posits the existence
of objective moral facts and values, while moral anti-realism denies their
existence. Cognitivism views moral judgments as expressions of beliefs
that can be true or false. Normative ethics establishes moral norms and
principles for ethical behavior in bioethical contexts, with consequentialist and deontological theories being commonly used. Natural law
theory and virtue ethics also play a role in guiding ethical decision-making in bioethics.

Ethics is not about Sexual behavior

One's sexuality is not what defines ethical behavior. In the field of bioethics, the focus is not primarily on sexuality and sexual behavior due to the broader scope of ethical considerations and the diverse range of moral issues that bioethicists address. While sexuality and sexual behavior are important aspects of human life and health, bioethics encompasses a wide array of ethical dilemmas and principles that extend beyond individual behaviors. Despite the importance of sexuality in human life and health, bioethical inquiries into sexual behavior have been limited. Wahlert & Fiester (2011) highlight that bioethical inquiries on sexuality and gender identity have been understudied, despite the pressing and sensitive issues faced by a significant and marginalized segment of the clinical population. Hedgecoe (2009) emphasizes that bioethics primarily addresses ethical problems raised by new technologies and medical practices, such as human cloning and stem cell research, rather than focusing on sexual behavior. Additionally, Wahlert and Fiester Wahlert & Fiester (2014) advocate for a new approach to bioethics, termed queer bioethics, which considers the perspectives, histories, and feelings of LGBT individuals in healthcare settings.

Bioethics often centers on complex ethical issues related to healthcare, medical research, end-of-life care, patient rights, informed consent, genetic testing, organ donation, resource allocation, and the use of emerging technologies in medicine. These areas raise critical ethical questions about patient autonomy, beneficence, nonmaleficence, justice, and the ethical responsibilities of healthcare professionals and institutions. References such as the European Resuscitation Council Guidelines 2021 on the ethics of resuscitation and end-of-life decisions, the reconceptualization of autonomy in bioethics, and discussions on the ethics of artificial intelligence in pathology highlight the diverse ethical challenges and considerations that bioethicists engage in within their work.

Ethics is not about Codes of Behavior

Codes of behavior, such as actions towards others, adultery, and theft, are not the primary sources of bioethics due to the broader scope of ethical considerations within the field. Bioethics encompasses a wide range of ethical dilemmas and principles that extend beyond individual behaviors. While codes of behavior may address specific actions or moral guidelines, bioethics delves into complex ethical issues related to healthcare, medical research, patient rights, informed consent, end-of-life care, genetic testing, organ donation, and the use of technology in medicine. These areas raise critical ethical questions about patient autonomy, beneficence, non-maleficence, justice, and the ethical responsibilities of healthcare professionals and institutions. Bioethics focuses on the ethical implications of healthcare practices, research, and policies, addressing a diverse array of moral issues that extend beyond individual behaviors or actions outlined in codes of behavior.

The "do unto others" golden rule, a fundamental ethical principle, holds significant relevance in the world of ethical theories. This principle, often associated with empathy, reciprocity, and moral conduct, transcends cultural and religious boundaries, serving as a universal guideline for ethical behavior. The verse commonly known as the Golden Rule in the Bible can be found in Matthew 7:12, where Jesus states, "All things therefore which you will that people do to you, do thus to them for this is the law and the prophets" (Carson, 2013). This verse encapsulates the principle of treating others as you would like to be treated, emphasizing empathy, compassion, and fairness in human interactions. The Golden Rule serves as a moral guideline for believers, encouraging them to act with kindness and consideration towards others. This biblical teaching has transcended religious boundaries and has been recognized as a universal moral value (Kinnier et al., 2000). It promotes virtues such as respect, compassion, truthfulness, justice, personal responsibility, self-discipline, courage, and faith. The Golden Rule is not only a religious precept but also a fundamental principle that underpins prosocial behavior and ethical conduct in various contexts (Slater & Banakou, 2021). While the Golden Rule is often associated with Christianity, its essence can be found in other cultures and belief systems, highlighting its universal appeal and relevance in promoting harmonious relationships and societal well-being. The verse from Matthew 7:12 continues to inspire individuals to practice empathy and consideration towards others, fostering a sense of interconnectedness and mutual respect in diverse communities.

In the realm of ethical theories, the golden rule embodies the concept of treating others with respect, compassion, and fairness, reflecting a fundamental moral duty to consider the well-being and interests of others as one's own. This principle aligns with various ethical frameworks, emphasizing the importance of empathy, reciprocity, and ethical conduct in interpersonal relationships, decision-making, and societal interactions. In ethical theories, the golden rule serves as a guiding principle for promoting moral behavior, fostering empathy and understanding, and cultivating a sense of shared humanity and ethical responsibility towards others.

Ethics is not just about Religion

Bioethics transcends religion by providing a framework for ethical decision-making that is inclusive of diverse cultural, religious, and philosophical perspectives. While religious beliefs and teachings may inform individual ethical viewpoints, bioethics as a field aims to address ethical dilemmas in healthcare, research, and public health in a way that is accessible and relevant to individuals of all faiths and beliefs. By drawing on principles such as autonomy, beneficence, nonmaleficence, and justice, bioethics offers a common ethical language that can be applied universally, regardless of religious affiliation. This approach allows for ethical discourse that is respectful of diverse beliefs and values, fostering dialogue, understanding, and collaboration in addressing complex ethical issues in healthcare and biomedical research. Bioethics provides a secular and inclusive ethical framework that promotes ethical decision-making based on reason, evidence, and the well-being of individuals and communities while respecting the diversity of religious and cultural perspectives.

In Judaism, Christianity, and Islam, there are specific religious teachings and principles that regulate bioethical discussions and guide ethical decision-making in various healthcare contexts. Here are examples from each of these religious traditions:

Judaism and Bioethics

In Judaism, the concept of "pikuach nefesh" (saving a life) is a fundamental principle that prioritizes the preservation of life above all else. This principle influences bioethical discussions related to medical interventions, organ donation, end-of-life care, and reproductive technologies. The Jewish tradition also emphasizes the importance of informed consent, patient autonomy, and the ethical considerations surrounding medical treatment and research. Rabbis and religious authorities play a role in interpreting Jewish law and guiding ethical decision-making in healthcare settings.

Judaism, like many other religions, plays a significant role in shaping bioethical perspectives and practices. In Judaism, various bioethical issues such as end-of-life care, assisted reproduction, xenotransplantation, euthanasia, and organ donation are influenced by traditional viewpoints and religious teachings (Cohen et al., 2008). For instance, Judaism generally permits the practice of assisted reproduction techniques as long as the biological materials come from the wife and husband (Schenker, 2005). Moreover, Jewish bioethics, rooted in principles derived from Jewish law (Halakhah), offers a unique perspective on bioethical dilemmas, even for those who do not share the same religious beliefs (Mathieu, 2016). The Jewish perspective on bioethics is not monolithic, as there exist diverse opinions within Judaism regarding issues like euthanasia (Baeke et al., 2011). The methodology of Jewish ethical reasoning and the diversity of thought within Judaism contribute to a rich discourse on bioethical matters (Baeke et al., 2011).

Furthermore, Jewish bioethics is deeply intertwined with religious texts and teachings, such as the Torah and Talmud, which provide guidance on ethical decision-making in various medical and healthcare contexts (Tarabeih, 2023). In the realm of end-of-life care, Jewish bio-ethical perspectives emphasize the importance of accountability before God and quality of life constructs, reflecting the values and beliefs of the Jewish faith (Padela & Mohiuddin, 2015). Additionally, Jewish bioethics engages with modern advancements in science and technology, such as synthetic biology, offering a Jewish approach to addressing the ethical implications of emerging technologies (Glick, 2012). Overall, Jewish bioethics is a dynamic field that draws from centuries-old religious traditions and texts to provide ethical guidance on contemporary medical and healthcare issues. By integrating religious teachings with modern ethical frameworks, Judaism contributes a unique and valuable perspective to the broader discourse on bioethics.

Christianity and Bioethics

In Christianity, the sanctity of life is a central ethical principle that informs bioethical discussions on issues such as abortion, euthanasia, and end-of-life care. The belief in the inherent value and dignity of every human life shapes ethical considerations in medical decision-making. Christian teachings on compassion, mercy, and the duty to care for the sick influence ethical discussions about healthcare practices, patient rights, and healthcare providers' ethical responsibilities.

Christianity has a significant influence on bioethics principles, particularly in the context of medical decision-making and patient care. The compatibility of values such as integrity, charity, and informed consent with ethical considerations surrounding practices like organ transplantation is evident (Priambodo, 2022). Christian teachings emphasize the moral imperative to care for patients and alleviate suffering, resonating with values of compassion and service (Delaney, 2021). Christian bioethics is deeply rooted in religious virtues and spiritual practices. The debate on whether Christian bioethics should be approached as a human activity grounded in theological study or as a result of spiritual disciplines leading to an encounter with God highlights the multifaceted nature of ethical considerations within a Christian framework (Cherry, 2020). The sanctity of human life, a fundamental principle in Judeo-Christian tradition, underpins bioethical discussions and decision-making processes (Maestre, 2018). The Incarnation, a central Christian doctrine, guides Christian bioethics, emphasizing the embodiment of ethical values in practical applications (Waters, 2005). Christian traditions, including Calvinist theology, provide resources for addressing modern bioethical challenges, showcasing the ongoing relevance of religious perspectives in bioethical discourse (Rocha, 2018). Christianity's influence extends to end-of-life care decisions, where religious affiliation plays a crucial role in medical decision-making, reflecting the significance of spiritual beliefs in shaping ethical considerations (Kassim & Alias, 2015). The belief in the sanctity of life, influenced by monotheistic faith perspectives, guides approaches to complex bioethical dilemmas, emphasizing the value of life and autonomy in healthcare decision-making (Khan et al., 2012).

Islam and Bioethics

In Islam, the concept of "fiqh al-mu'amalat" (Islamic jurisprudence in transactions) guides ethical decision-making in various aspects of life, including healthcare. Islamic bioethics emphasizes principles such as respect for life, beneficence, nonmaleficence, and justice in medical practice. Islamic teachings on the sanctity of life, the duty to care for the sick, and the importance of ethical conduct shape bioethical discussions on issues such as organ donation, end-of-life care, and medical research.

Islamic bioethics is a framework guided by fundamental principles rooted in Islamic law, known as Shari'ah. These principles dictate that all ethical rulings and actions must align with Islamic teachings, emphasizing the importance of adhering to the Qur'an and the teachings of Prophet Muhammad (Chamsi-Pasha & Albar, 2015). Islamic bioethics is an extension of Shari'ah, which is based on the Qur'an and the Sunnah, aiming to identify, analyze, and resolve ethical dilemmas in medical practice and research (Woodman et al., 2022). Islamic bioethics places significant emphasis on the sanctity of life, seeking treatment, and preserving life, reflecting the core values of compassion and care within Islamic teachings (Chandrasekar et al., 2022). The ethical framework in Islam is deeply intertwined with religious and ethical considerations, with a focus on the interconnectedness between the material and spiritual realms (Salter, 2021). Islamic bioethics is grounded in textual references, making it a blend of religious and ethical perspectives (Muhsin, 2021). In addressing bioethical issues, Islamic scholars have introduced principles such as "the Public Interest," "Do no Harm," "Necessity," and "No Hardship" to guide ethical judgments in medical contexts (Farajkhoda, 2017). These principles provide a basis for evaluating and resolving ethical dilemmas in medical practice and research, aligning with Islamic moral and legislative sources (Woodman et al., 2022). Islamic bioethics also encompasses the application of ethical values to specific medical contexts, such as genetic counseling and reproductive health services. Scholars have developed frameworks within Islamic bioethics to justify regulations on access to key reproductive health services for at-risk adolescents, highlighting the ongoing development and adaptation of ethical principles to contemporary healthcare challenges (Akrami et al., 2022).

Meta-ethics Theory

Meta-ethics in bioethics refers to the study of the nature, scope, and foundations of ethical principles and theories. It delves into questions about the meaning of ethical terms, the nature of moral judgments, and the relationship between facts and values in ethical reasoning. Meta-ethics explores the underlying assumptions and concepts that inform ethical theories and helps to clarify the philosophical basis of ethical discourse in bioethics. In bioethics, meta-ethics is a critical field that delves into the fundamental aspects of ethical principles and theories within the context of biomedical practices and research. This branch of ethics focuses on examining the nature, scope, and foundations of ethical principles and theories that guide decision-making in the realm of bioethics. Meta-ethics in bioethics is concerned with elucidating the meaning of ethical terms, understanding the nature of moral judgments, and exploring the intricate relationship between facts and values in ethical reasoning. One of the central inquiries in meta-ethics is the examination of the underlying assumptions and concepts that underpin ethical theories. By scrutinizing these foundational elements, researchers and scholars aim to gain a deeper understanding of the philosophical basis of ethical discourse in bioethics. This process involves critically analyzing the various ethical frameworks and principles that are applied in the field of bioethics, such as autonomy, beneficence, non-maleficence, and justice. Moreover, meta-ethics in bioethics plays a vital role in clarifying the ethical landscape within the realm of biomedicine. It helps to identify and address key ethical dilemmas and challenges that arise in clinical practice, research, and healthcare policy. By engaging in meta-ethical analysis, bioethicists can better navigate complex ethical issues, resolve moral conflicts, and develop ethically sound guidelines and recommendations for ethical decision-making in healthcare settings. Furthermore, meta-ethics in bioethics contributes to the ongoing dialogue surrounding the ethical implications of advances in biotechnology, genetics, and medical interventions. Scholars in this field can offer valuable insights into the ethical considerations associated with emerging technologies and scientific developments in biomedicine by examining the nature of moral judgments and the relationship between facts and values in ethical reasoning.

Normative Ethics Theory

Normative ethics theories in bioethics, on the other hand, focus on determining what actions are morally right or wrong in specific situations. These theories provide frameworks for evaluating ethical dilemmas, making moral judgments, and guiding ethical decision-making in healthcare and biomedical research.

Normative ethics theories, such as consequentialism, deontology, virtue ethics, and principlism, offer different perspectives on how to determine the ethical course of action in bioethical contexts. By examining meta-ethics and normative ethics theories in bioethics, scholars and practitioners can gain a deeper understanding of the philosophical underpinnings of ethical principles, the nature of moral reasoning, and the application of ethical theories in healthcare practice and research. These theoretical perspectives help to inform ethical discussions, guide ethical decision-making, and promote ethical conduct in the field of bioethics.

Normative ethics theories in bioethics serve as essential tools for evaluating and determining the moral rightness or wrongness of actions within specific contexts in healthcare and biomedical research. These theories offer structured frameworks that aid in navigating ethical dilemmas, making moral judgments, and providing guidance for ethical decision-making processes. Consequentialism, a prominent normative ethics theory, posits that the morality of an action is determined by its outcomes or consequences. Utilitarianism, a specific form of consequentialism, emphasizes maximizing overall happiness or well-being as the ethical goal.

Deontology, another significant normative ethics theory, focuses on the inherent moral principles or duties that should guide actions, regardless of their consequences. Virtue ethics, on the other hand, emphasizes the development of virtuous character traits and habits as central to ethical decision-making. Principlism, a widely used approach in bioethics, involves the application of key ethical principles such as autonomy, beneficence, non-maleficence, and justice to ethical dilemmas in healthcare. By integrating meta-ethics and normative ethics theories in bioethics, scholars and practitioners can deepen their understanding of the philosophical foundations of ethical principles and the nature of moral reasoning. Meta-ethics provides the groundwork for examining the underlying assumptions and concepts that inform normative ethics theories, while normative ethics theories offer practical guidance on how to assess and address ethical challenges in healthcare settings. The application of normative ethics theories in bioethics facilitates ethical discussions, informs decision-making processes, and fosters ethical behavior among healthcare professionals and researchers. By engaging with these theoretical perspectives, individuals involved in bioethics can navigate complex ethical issues, uphold ethical standards, and promote the well-being of patients and research participants.

Moral Realism

Moral realism is a meta-ethical theory that posits the existence of objective moral facts and values that are independent of individual beliefs, opinions, or cultural norms. According to moral realism, moral truths are objective and universal, existing in the world as real properties that can be discovered and known. This perspective suggests that moral statements can be true or false, and moral judgments are based on an external reality rather than subjective preferences or social conventions. Moral realism asserts that there are moral facts that are true regardless of human beliefs or attitudes, providing a foundation for ethical objectivity and moral knowledge in bioethics and other ethical domains.

Moral realism is a meta-ethical theory that stands in contrast to moral anti-realism, which denies the existence of objective moral truths. Moral realism posits that there are objective moral facts and values that exist independently of individual beliefs, opinions, or cultural norms. This perspective asserts that moral truths are not merely subjective constructs but are inherent properties of the world that can be discovered and known through ethical inquiry. Central to moral realism is the idea that moral statements have truth value and can be objectively true or false. This implies that ethical judgments are not solely based on personal preferences or societal conventions but are grounded in an external reality that transcends individual perspectives. Proponents of moral realism argue that there are moral facts that hold true regardless of human beliefs or attitudes, providing a basis for ethical objectivity and moral knowledge. In the context of bioethics and other ethical domains, moral realism offers a framework for understanding and evaluating ethical principles and dilemmas. By positing the existence of objective moral facts, moral realism supports the notion that ethical decisions can be based on universal standards rather than subjective interpretations. This has significant implications for ethical discourse and decision-making in fields such as healthcare, where moral considerations play a crucial role in guiding practices and policies. Moreover, moral realism provides a foundation for ethical objectivity, emphasizing the importance of recognizing and adhering to moral truths that exist independently of individual perspectives. This perspective underscores the idea that ethical principles are not mere social constructs but are rooted in an objective reality that transcends cultural variations and personal beliefs. Overall, moral realism contributes to the philosophical underpinnings of bioethics by asserting the existence of objective moral facts and values. Moral realism enriches ethical discourse by acknowledging the presence of universal moral truths, promotes ethical objectivity, and enhances our understanding of ethical principles and decision-making processes in bioethics and beyond.

Moral Anti-Realism

Moral anti-realism is a meta-ethical position that denies the existence of objective moral facts or values. Moral statements do not correspond to objective truths or properties in the world, according to moral anti-realism. Instead, moral judgments are considered to be subjective, relative, or culturally dependent, lacking universal validity or truth. Moral anti-realism encompasses various sub-positions, such as moral relativism, moral subjectivism, and error theory, which challenge the idea of objective moral truths and question the possibility of moral knowledge that is independent of individual beliefs or cultural norms. In bioethics, moral anti-realism raises questions about the nature of moral values, the objectivity of ethical principles, and the foundations of moral reasoning, challenging traditional views of moral objectivity and universal moral truths.

Moral Anti-Realism Moral anti-realism is a meta-ethical position that denies the existence of objective moral facts or values. Moral statements do not correspond to objective truths or properties in the world, according to moral anti-realism. Instead, moral judgments are considered to be subjective, relative, or culturally dependent, lacking universal validity or truth. Moral anti-realism encompasses various sub-positions, such as moral relativism, moral subjectivism, and error theory, which challenge the idea of objective moral truths and question the possibility of moral knowledge that is independent of individual beliefs or cultural norms. In bioethics, moral anti-realism raises questions about the nature of moral values, the objectivity of ethical principles, and the foundations of moral reasoning, challenging traditional views of moral objectivity and universal moral truths.

Moral anti-realism represents a significant meta-ethical stance that challenges the existence of objective moral facts or values. This position asserts that moral statements lack correspondence to any objective truths or properties in the world, thereby rejecting the notion of universal moral validity. Instead, moral anti-realism posits that moral judgments are subjective, relative, or culturally contingent, devoid of universal truth or validity. This perspective encompasses various sub-positions, including moral relativism, moral subjectivism, and error theory, each of which contributes to skepticism towards the existence of objective moral truths. Moral relativism, a form of moral anti-realism, argues that moral judgments are context-dependent and vary across different cultures or societies. It suggests that there are no universal moral standards that apply to all individuals or communities, emphasizing the diversity of moral beliefs and practices. Moral subjectivism, another sub-position within moral anti-realism, contends that moral judgments are grounded in individual attitudes, emotions, or preferences rather than objective moral facts. According to moral subjectivism, ethical principles are subjective constructs that reflect personal perspectives and values. Error theory, a further sub-position of moral anti-realism, posits that moral statements are systematically mistaken due to the lack of objective moral truths. Error theorists argue that moral language is fundamentally flawed, as it presupposes the existence of moral facts that do not align with reality. This perspective challenges the possibility of moral knowledge that is independent of individual beliefs or cultural norms, casting doubt on the foundations of moral reasoning and ethical discourse. In the realm of bioethics, moral anti-realism raises profound questions about the nature of moral values, the objectivity of ethical principles, and the basis of moral reasoning. By rejecting the existence of objective moral truths, moral anti-realism challenges traditional views of moral objectivity and universal moral principles that have historically guided ethical decision-making in healthcare and biomedical research. This critical perspective prompts scholars and practitioners in bioethics to engage in nuanced discussions about the relativity of moral values, the diversity of ethical perspectives, and the implications of moral anti-realism for ethical theory and practice in the field.

Cognitivism

Cognitivism in bioethics refers to the meta-ethical view that moral judgments and ethical statements express beliefs that can be true or false. This perspective holds that ethical claims are cognitive propositions that convey factual information about moral values and principles. Cognitivism asserts that ethical language has cognitive content and can be understood in terms of truth and falsity, distinguishing it from non-cognitive or emotivist views that see moral statements as expressions of emotions or attitudes. In bioethics, cognitivism provides a framework for analyzing and evaluating ethical arguments, theories, and principles based on their truth value and rational justification.

Cognitivism in bioethics represents a meta-ethical position that views moral judgments and ethical statements as expressions of beliefs that can be objectively true or false. This perspective asserts that ethical claims are cognitive propositions that convey factual information about moral values and principles, suggesting that ethical language carries cognitive content that can be analyzed in terms of truth and falsity. Cognitivism stands in contrast to non-cognitive views, such as emotivism, which interpret moral statements as mere expressions of emotions or attitudes without inherent truth value. In the context of bioethics, cognitivism offers a structured framework for examining and assessing ethical arguments, theories, and principles based on their truth value and rational justification. By treating ethical statements as propositions that can be evaluated for their truth or falsity, cognitivism enables scholars and practitioners in bioethics to engage in critical analysis and reasoned debate regarding ethical issues in healthcare and biomedical research. Cognitivism in bioethics facilitates a deeper understanding of the cognitive content of ethical language, emphasizing the importance of rational discourse and logical reasoning in ethical decision-making processes. This perspective emphasizes the role of moral beliefs as truth-apt propositions that can be scrutinized and evaluated based on objective criteria. Moreover, cognitivism provides a basis for ethical discourse that is grounded in reasoned argumentation and evidence-based reasoning. By recognizing ethical claims as statements that can be true or false, cognitivism encourages a more rigorous and systematic approach to ethical analysis, fostering clarity and precision in ethical discussions within the field of bioethics. Overall, cognitivism in bioethics enriches ethical inquiry by emphasizing the cognitive nature of moral judgments and ethical statements. By acknowledging the truth-apt status of ethical propositions, cognitivism contributes to the development of a robust ethical framework that promotes critical thinking, logical analysis, and informed decision-making in the complex and multifaceted domain of bioethics.

Normative Ethics

Normative ethics in bioethics refers to the branch of ethics that is concerned with establishing the moral norms, principles, and guidelines that govern ethical behavior and decision-making in healthcare, biomedical research, and related fields. Normative ethics provides a framework for evaluating the rightness or wrongness of actions, determining ethical duties and obligations, and guiding ethical conduct in bioethical contexts. This branch of ethics addresses questions about what actions are morally permissible, required, or forbidden in specific situations, and it offers ethical theories and principles that inform ethical decision-making and practice in healthcare settings. Normative ethics in bioethics plays a crucial role in shaping ethical standards, promoting ethical behavior, and addressing complex ethical dilemmas that arise in the field of healthcare and biomedical research.

Normative ethics in bioethics serves as a foundational pillar in the realm of ethical inquiry, focusing on the establishment of moral norms, principles, and guidelines that govern ethical conduct and decision-making within healthcare, biomedical research, and related domains. This branch of ethics provides a structured framework for assessing the moral implications of actions, delineating ethical duties and responsibilities, and offering guidance on ethical behavior in bioethical contexts. Normative ethics addresses fundamental questions concerning the moral permissibility, obligation, or prohibition of actions in specific situations within the healthcare and biomedical spheres. By drawing upon various ethical theories and principles, normative ethics offers a toolkit for evaluating ethical dilemmas, resolving moral conflicts, and navigating complex ethical challenges that arise in clinical practice, research, and healthcare policy. The application of normative ethics in bioethics is instrumental in shaping ethical standards and fostering a culture of ethical behavior among healthcare professionals, researchers, and policymakers. By providing a framework for ethical decision-making, normative ethics helps to ensure that actions taken in healthcare settings align with established moral norms and principles, promoting integrity, trust, and accountability in the delivery of healthcare services and the conduct of biomedical research. Moreover, normative ethics plays a pivotal role in addressing ethical dilemmas that are inherent to the field of bioethics, such as issues related to patient autonomy, end-of-life care, genetic testing, and resource allocation. By offering ethical theories and principles that guide ethical reasoning and practice, normative ethics equips individuals involved in bioethics with the tools necessary to navigate moral complexities, uphold ethical standards, and make ethically sound decisions that prioritize the well-being of patients, research participants, and the broader community.

Normative Ethics and Utilitarianism

Normative ethics theory, specifically utilitarianism, is a moral framework that evaluates the ethicality of actions based on their consequences, with the principle of maximizing overall happiness or utility. Utilitarianism posits that the right course of action is the one that produces the greatest amount of happiness or pleasure for the greatest number of people.

This ethical theory focuses on action outcomes and seeks to promote the greatest good for the greatest number, emphasizing the importance of considering the overall consequences of one's actions in ethical decision-making. Utilitarianism is a consequentialist theory that prioritizes the well-being and happiness of individuals and society as a whole, providing a framework for evaluating ethical dilemmas and guiding moral judgments in bioethical contexts.

Normative Ethics and Deontological Moral Theory

Normative ethics theory, specifically deontological moral theory, is a moral framework that emphasizes the inherent rightness or wrongness of actions themselves rather than focusing solely on their consequences. Deontological ethics is based on the idea that certain actions are intrinsically moral or immoral, regardless of their outcomes. This ethical theory is often associated with the philosopher Immanuel Kant and his concept of the categorical imperative, which asserts that individuals have a moral duty to act in accordance with universal principles and moral laws. Deontological moral theory in bioethics provides a framework for evaluating ethical dilemmas and making moral judgments based on principles of duty, obligation, and moral rules. This approach prioritizes the intention behind actions, the adherence to moral principles, and the inherent moral worth of certain actions, rather than solely focusing on the consequences of those actions. Deontological ethics offers a perspective that emphasizes the importance of moral duties, rights, and principles in guiding ethical decision-making and behavior in healthcare, biomedical research, and other bioethical contexts.

Normative ethics, particularly deontological moral theory, offers a distinctive ethical framework that places emphasis on the intrinsic rightness or wrongness of actions themselves rather than solely considering their outcomes. Deontological ethics is rooted in the notion that certain actions possess inherent moral value or lack thereof, irrespective of the consequences they may yield. This ethical perspective is closely associated with the philosopher Immanuel Kant and his formulation of the categorical imperative, which posits that individuals have a moral obligation to act in accordance with universal moral principles and laws that are binding on all rational beings. Deontological moral theory in bioethics provides a structured approach for evaluating ethical dilemmas and making moral judgments based on principles of duty, obligation, and moral rules. This ethical framework prioritizes the intention behind actions, the adherence to moral principles, and the intrinsic moral worth of certain actions. By focusing on the moral duties and obligations that individuals have towards others and society, deontological ethics offers a principled perspective that guides ethical decision-making in healthcare, biomedical research, and various bioethical contexts. The emphasis on moral duties and principles in deontological ethics underscores the significance of acting in accordance with ethical norms and rules, regardless of the consequences that may ensue. This approach highlights the importance of upholding moral principles and fulfilling one's duties and obligations as essential components of ethical behavior. By prioritizing the intention behind actions and the adherence to moral rules, deontological ethics provides a robust ethical framework that promotes moral integrity, respect for individual rights, and the pursuit of moral excellence in bioethical practice. In the realm of bioethics, deontological moral theory offers valuable insights into ethical decision-making processes, guiding practitioners and policymakers to consider the moral principles and duties that underpin their actions. By emphasizing the significance of moral rules, rights, and obligations, deontological ethics contributes to the cultivation of a morally responsible healthcare environment that upholds ethical standards, respects individual autonomy, and prioritizes the well-being of patients and research participants.

Normative Ethics and Natural Law Theory

Normative ethics theory, specifically natural law theory, is a moral framework that posits the existence of universal moral principles derived from nature or reason. According to natural law theory, there are inherent moral truths that are discoverable through human reason and applicable to all individuals, regardless of cultural or religious beliefs. This ethical theory emphasizes the importance of aligning human actions with these objective moral principles to promote ethical behavior and societal harmony. Natural law theory provides a foundation for ethical decision-making in bioethics, guiding individuals and healthcare professionals in determining right and wrong actions based on universal moral principles derived from nature or reason.

Normative ethics, particularly natural law theory, offers a moral framework that asserts the existence of universal moral principles that are inherent in nature or discernible through human reason. Natural law theory posits that there are objective moral truths that are rooted in the natural order and can be discovered through rational reflection. These moral principles are considered to be binding on all individuals, transcending cultural, religious, or societal differences. Natural law theory's ethical perspective emphasizes the importance of aligning human actions with these universal moral principles to foster ethical conduct and societal well-being. In the realm of bioethics, natural law theory serves as a foundational basis for ethical decision-making, providing a framework for individuals and healthcare professionals to discern right from wrong based on universal moral principles derived from nature or reason. By emphasizing the importance of adhering to objective moral truths that are inherent in the natural order, natural law theory guides ethical behavior and decision-making processes in healthcare, biomedical research, and related bioethical contexts. Natural law theory highlights the notion that ethical norms are not arbitrary or culturally contingent but are grounded in the inherent order of the natural world. This perspective suggests that there are fundamental moral principles that govern human conduct and can be ascertained through rational inquiry and reflection. By aligning human actions with these universal moral principles, individuals are encouraged to uphold ethical standards, promote human flourishing, and contribute to the common good. In the context of bioethics, natural law theory offers a principled approach to addressing ethical dilemmas and navigating complex moral issues. By drawing on the concept of universal moral principles derived from nature or reason, natural law theory provides a robust ethical framework that guides ethical decision-making, promotes moral integrity, and fosters a deeper understanding of the ethical dimensions of healthcare practices and biomedical research. This ethical perspective underscores the importance of aligning human actions with objective moral truths to uphold ethical standards and advance the well-being of individuals as well as society as a whole.

Normative Ethics and Virtue Ethics

Normative ethics and virtue ethics are two branches of ethical theory that play a significant role in guiding moral decision-making and behavior in various contexts, including bioethics. Normative ethics focuses on determining the moral standards and principles that govern right and wrong actions, providing a framework for evaluating ethical dilemmas and making moral judgments. On the other hand, virtue ethics emphasizes the development of moral character, virtues, and personal qualities that lead to ethical behavior and flourishing. In bioethics, normative ethics theories help to establish ethical guidelines and principles that inform healthcare practices, research, and decision-making processes. These theories provide a framework for assessing the ethical implications of medical interventions, patient care, and biomedical research. Virtue ethics, on the other hand, emphasizes the importance of cultivating virtues such as compassion, integrity, empathy, and honesty in healthcare professionals to promote ethical conduct and enhance patient care. By integrating normative ethics and virtue ethics in bioethics, practitioners and scholars can address ethical challenges, promote ethical behavior, and uphold moral values in healthcare settings. These ethical theories offer complementary perspectives on ethical decision-making, emphasizing both the principles that guide moral actions and the virtues that shape ethical character and conduct in the field of bioethics.

Normative ethics and virtue ethics represent two distinct branches of ethical theory that contribute significantly to the ethical landscape, particularly in the realm of bioethics. Normative ethics is concerned with establishing the moral standards and principles that govern right and wrong actions, providing a structured framework for evaluating ethical dilemmas, and making moral judgments. In contrast, virtue ethics places emphasis on the cultivation of moral character, virtues, and personal qualities that lead to ethical behavior and human flourishing. In the context of bioethics, normative ethics theories serve as a foundation for establishing ethical guidelines and principles that inform healthcare practices, research endeavors, and decision-making processes. These theories offer a systematic approach to assessing the ethical implications of medical interventions, patient care, and biomedical research, guiding practitioners and policymakers in navigating complex ethical issues and dilemmas that arise in healthcare settings. Virtue ethics, on the other hand, underscores the importance of developing virtuous character traits such as compassion, integrity, empathy, and honesty in healthcare professionals. By focusing on the cultivation of virtues that shape ethical character and conduct, virtue ethics aims to promote ethical behavior, enhance patient care, and foster a culture of moral excellence within healthcare environments. The integration of normative ethics and virtue ethics in bioethics allows for a comprehensive approach to addressing ethical challenges, promoting ethical conduct, and upholding moral values in healthcare settings. By combining the principles and guidelines provided by normative ethics theories with the emphasis on character development and virtues advocated by virtue ethics, practitioners and scholars in bioethics can navigate ethical dilemmas with a holistic perspective that considers both the ethical principles guiding actions and the moral virtues shaping ethical character. Overall, normative ethics and virtue ethics offer complementary perspectives on ethical decision-making in bioethics, highlighting the importance of both ethical principles and virtuous character traits in promoting ethical behavior, enhancing patient care, and fostering a culture of integrity and compassion within the healthcare field.

TERMINOLOGY

1. **Autonomy** - A principle in bioethics that upholds the right of individuals to make informed decisions about their own healthcare based on personal values and beliefs.

2. **Beneficence** - The ethical principle that involves acting in the best interests of others, which in healthcare includes promoting the well-being of patients and taking actions that will benefit them.

3. **Bioethics** - A field of study that addresses ethical issues and dilemmas arising from advances in biology and medicine, including healthcare, medical research, and technology.

4. **Cognitivism** - A meta-ethical view that asserts moral judgments are expressions of beliefs that can be true or false, and that ethical statements convey factual information about moral values.

5. **Consequentialism** - An ethical theory that judges the rightness or wrongness of actions solely by their consequences. The most well-known form, utilitarianism, advocates for actions that maximize overall happiness or well-being.

6. **Deontology** - An ethical theory that focuses on the inherent moral duties and rules that should guide behavior, emphasizing that some actions are morally right or wrong regardless of their outcomes.

7. **Error Theory** - A sub-position within moral anti-realism that suggests moral statements are systematically flawed as they often assume the existence of objective moral truths that do not actually exist.

8. **Fiqh al-mu'amalat** - In Islam, jurisprudence dealing with ethical decision-making in transactions and everyday life, impacting discussions in medical ethics about care and treatment.

9. **Justice** - In bioethics, the principle that emphasizes fairness in the distribution of resources and respect for people's rights, ensuring equitable treatment in healthcare settings.

10. **Meta-ethics** - A branch of ethics that explores the nature, scope, and meaning of ethical terms and judgments, focusing on the underlying philosophical aspects of moral thought.

11. **Moral Anti-Realism** - A meta-ethical stance arguing that there are no objective moral facts, with moral values being subjective or culturally dependent.

12. **Moral Realism** - The belief in meta-ethics that moral truths exist independently of human perception, and that objective moral facts can guide ethical decision-making.

13. **Natural Law Theory** - An ethical framework that posits the existence of universal moral principles derived from nature and discernible through reason, guiding human conduct and ethical decisions.

14. **Nonmaleficence** - A fundamental principle in healthcare ethics that entails not inflicting harm on others, guiding medical professionals in their practice and decision-making.

15. **Normative Ethics** - The study of ethical action. It investigates the set of questions that arise when considering how one ought to act, morally speaking.

16. **Pikuach Nefesh** - A principle in Jewish bioethics prioritizing the preservation and sanctity of human life, often guiding decisions in medical ethics regarding life-saving interventions.

17. **Principlism** - An approach in bioethics that uses key ethical principles, such as autonomy, beneficence, non-maleficence, and justice, to resolve ethical dilemmas in healthcare.

18. **Relativism** - A theory within moral anti-realism suggesting that moral principles and values are relative to specific cultural or individual contexts.

19. **Sanctity of Life** - A belief in the inherent value and dignity of all human lives, often influencing bioethical discussions on topics like euthanasia and end-of-life care.

20. **Shari'ah** - Islamic law derived from the Quran and the Hadith, influencing Islamic bioethics and guiding ethical decision-making in healthcare among Muslims.

21. **Subjectivism** - A branch of moral anti-realism which posits that moral judgments and ethical principles are based on personal feelings, attitudes, or opinions, rather than objective truths.

22. **Utilitarianism** - A consequentialist ethical theory that determines the rightness of actions based on their outcomes, specifically the overall happiness or well-being they produce.

23. **Virtue Ethics** - An ethical theory that emphasizes the role of character and virtue in moral philosophy rather than either the consequences of actions or the rules governing them.

DISCUSSION QUESTIONS:

1. **Autonomy vs. Public Health:**

   Scenario: Imagine a scenario where a highly contagious disease is spreading rapidly. A vaccine is available, but many citizens refuse vaccination based on personal belief. Should the government mandate vaccinations to protect public health, or should individual autonomy be respected? How do different ethical theories inform your decision?

2. **Genetic Testing and Privacy:**

   Scenario: Consider a world where employers can access the genetic information of potential employees. A company learns about a candidate's genetic predisposition to a severe mental health disorder and decides not to hire them based on this information. Is this decision ethically justified? Discuss using principles of beneficence, nonmaleficence, and justice.

3. **Resource Allocation in Healthcare:**

   Scenario: A small island nation has a limited amount of a life-saving drug and must decide whether to prioritize the elderly or children for treatment. Which group should receive the drug first, and why? Discuss using consequentialist and deontological perspectives.

4. **Artificial Intelligence in Medicine:**

   Scenario: An AI system can accurately predict patient outcomes based on their symptoms and medical history, sometimes suggesting end-of-life care over treatment. Should doctors follow the AI recommendations, or should they consider other factors? What does virtue ethics have to say about this scenario?

5. **Organ Donation by Default:**

   Scenario: In a certain country, everyone is considered an organ donor unless they opt out. Some religious groups feel this policy infringes on their beliefs. How should the government address this issue? Discuss the balance between community benefit and respect for religious beliefs using natural law theory and moral realism.

6. **End-of-Life Decisions:**

   Scenario: A patient with a terminal illness requests euthanasia to end their suffering, but their family is vehemently opposed. Should the healthcare provider honor the patient's request? How does the principle of autonomy compete with the concept of sanctity of life in this scenario?

7. **Confidentiality vs. Potential Harm:**

   Scenario: A therapist learns that their patient, who works as a bus driver, has a medical condition that could potentially cause sudden unconsciousness but has not informed their employer.

Should the therapist break confidentiality to prevent potential harm? What would a moral anti-realist suggest?

8. **Queer Bioethics and Healthcare Discrimination:**

   Scenario: An LGBTQ+ patient experiences discrimination in a healthcare setting. The healthcare provider's personal beliefs about sexuality influence their treatment decisions. How should the hospital address this issue? Discuss using the perspectives of queer bioethics and the golden rule.

9. **Informed Consent in Culturally Diverse Settings:**

   Scenario: A medical trial is set up in a rural area where cultural beliefs about medicine differ significantly from the mainstream. Participants are wary of giving informed consent because they do not fully understand the medical jargon used. How should researchers ensure ethical practice? Discuss the implications using meta-ethics and cognitivism.

10. **Genetic Enhancement in Children:**

    Scenario: Parents can now choose genetic enhancements for their children, including increased intelligence and physical strength. Should there be limitations on these enhancements? Discuss the ethical implications using utilitarianism and deontological moral theory.

CHAPTER 3

MORAL NORMS

The term "ethics" encompasses various approaches to understanding moral behavior. Christian ethics plays a significant role in guiding ethical decision-making and shaping moral frameworks, particularly in the context of bioethics. The principles of sanctity of life, human dignity, compassion, and care, as well as justice and equity, are central to Christian ethics and common morality. The sanctity of life principle emphasizes the inherent value and dignity of every human life, guiding ethical considerations related to issues such as euthanasia, abortion, and end-of-life care. The principle of human dignity underscores the respect and worth of every individual, informing decisions regarding informed consent, patient autonomy, and the protection of vulnerable populations. Compassion and care are viewed as essential virtues that reflect the teachings of love, kindness, and empathy found in the Christian tradition, guiding healthcare providers in providing compassionate and patient-centered care. The principles of justice and equity promote fair treatment, access to care, and advocacy for marginalized populations, informing discussions on healthcare disparities, resource allocation, and social determinants of health. Individuals can navigate ethical dilemmas, promote individual and social well-being, and contribute to a more just and compassionate world by upholding these principles.

Normative Ethics

Normative ethics seeks to identify and justify the norms that should govern human conduct, while practical ethics applies these general moral norms to address specific issues. Normative ethics is a branch of ethics that aims to establish the principles and norms that should guide human behavior. It is concerned with determining what is morally right or wrong, good or bad, and just or unjust. Normative ethics provides a framework for evaluating actions and decisions based on ethical theories such as utilitarianism, deontology, virtue ethics, and ethical relativism. In the context of bioethics, normative ethics plays a crucial role in determining the moral norms that should govern practices related to human life, health, and well-being. Bioethics is a specialized field of ethics that deals with ethical issues arising in healthcare, biomedical research, and the life sciences. It involves applying ethical principles to dilemmas and controversies in areas such as medical treatment, genetic engineering, reproductive technologies, and end-of-life care. Moral norms in bioethics are derived from broader ethical theories and principles, but they are specifically tailored to address the complex and sensitive issues that arise in the context of healthcare and biotechnology. These norms help guide healthcare professionals, researchers, policymakers, and the general public in making ethically sound decisions and resolving moral conflicts in the realm of biomedicine.

To understand what it means to act morally right or wrong, good or bad, or just and unjust, we must delve into the realm of normative ethics. Normative ethics is concerned with establishing the principles and norms that should guide human behavior and decision-making. When an action is deemed morally right, it aligns with these established ethical norms and is considered to be in accordance with what is perceived as good, just, or right. Conversely, actions that are morally wrong go against these norms and are viewed as bad, unjust, or wrong. In the context of bioethics, which deals with ethical issues in healthcare and the life sciences, the concepts of right and wrong, good and bad, and just and unjust are crucial. For instance, in medical decision-making, it is essential to consider what actions are morally right in terms of providing the best care for patients, respecting their autonomy, and promoting beneficence and non-maleficence. Actions that deviate from these ethical principles may be considered morally wrong or unjust. Moreover, the idea of a just world plays a role in shaping moral beliefs and behaviors. People often have a fundamental need to believe in a just world where good actions are rewarded and bad actions are punished. This belief in a just world influences how individuals perceive and respond to moral dilemmas and injustices. It can also impact their judgments of what is morally right or wrong in a given situation. Normative ethics provides the framework for understanding what constitutes morally right or wrong, good or bad, and just or unjust behavior. These concepts are essential in guiding ethical decision-making in various fields, including bioethics, where adherence to moral norms is crucial for promoting the well-being and dignity of individuals.

Sources of moral good can be found in various texts and codes that shape ethical behavior and decision-making. These sources include religious texts, philosophical works, societal norms, and personal values. Religious texts such as the Bible, the Quran, or the Bhagavad Gita often provide moral guidelines and commandments that believers are expected to follow. These texts serve as sources of moral authority and influence the ethical beliefs and practices of individuals and communities (Koonce & Hyrkäs, 2022). Philosophical works by thinkers like Aristotle, Immanuel Kant, and John Stuart Mill offer ethical theories that provide insights into what constitutes moral goodness and how individuals should act ethically. For example, Kant's categorical imperative emphasizes the importance of acting from a sense of duty and following universal moral laws, while utilitarianism, advocated by Mill, focuses on maximizing overall happiness and well-being as a moral good (Cohen et al., 2006). Societal norms and codes of ethics also play a significant role in shaping moral behavior. Corporate codes of ethics, global codes of conduct, and business ethics literature contribute to defining universal moral values that guide ethical decision-making in the business world (Schwartz, 2005). Moreover, legal systems, parental guidance, peer influences, and cultural traditions all contribute to the formation of moral norms that influence individual behavior and societal standards of right and wrong (Branscum et al., 2022). Personal values and beliefs are another important source of moral goodness. Individuals often derive their sense of morality from their upbringing, education, and personal experiences. These internalized values guide their ethical choices and actions, reflecting their understanding of what is morally right or wrong (Smith & Masser, 2012).

Nonnormative Ethics

In addition to normative ethics, there are nonnormative ethics types. Nonnormative ethics refers to ethical theories or perspectives that do not rely on established norms or standards to determine what is morally right or wrong. Nonnormative ethics, instead of focusing on traditional moral principles, may explore alternative ethical approaches that do not conform to conventional moral frameworks. Nonnormative ethics can come from a variety of disciplines and perspectives that challenge or go beyond traditional normative ethical theories. A potential source of nonnormative ethics can be found in narrative entertainment and social psychology research. Studies that investigate the salience of moral intuitions through repeated exposure to narratives may offer insights into how individuals form moral judgments outside of normative ethical frameworks (Eden et al., 2014). By examining how moral intuitions are shaped by storytelling and social influences, researchers can explore nonnormative sources of ethical reasoning that may not align with established moral norms. Another source of nonnormative ethics could be the intersection of law and sustainable development. Legal conditions and principles related to sustainable development, as interpreted by the Court of Justice of the European Union, may provide a perspective on ethics that is not solely based on normative standards (Syryt & Klimska, 2019). By considering the legal norms and principles that underpin environmental protection and sustainable development, scholars can uncover ethical considerations that stem from legal frameworks rather than traditional moral norms. Furthermore, the field of mental health and disability studies may offer insights into nonnormative ethics by challenging conventional notions of normalcy and deviation. Analyzing how mental health conditions and disabilities are perceived and addressed in society can shed light on alternative ethical perspectives that do not adhere strictly to normative standards (Tsacoyianis, 2019). By exploring the experiences of individuals with nonnormative bodies or minds, researchers can uncover ethical considerations that extend beyond traditional moral frameworks.

Moral Norms

Descriptive ethics examines the actual moral beliefs and norms guiding human behavior, while metaethics analyzes the language, concepts, and reasoning methods in normative ethics. "Moral norms" refer to accepted standards of right and wrong behavior within a social context. Common morality consists of universally affirmed norms, obligations, and virtues. In contrast, particular moralities present specific, nonuniversal, and content-rich norms. Professions often adhere to professional moralities, reflected in codes of conduct like the American Medical Association's Code. Health professionals also receive moral guidance from government regulations and public policy.

Moral norms play a significant role in guiding human behavior and decision-making within social contexts. Descriptive ethics examines the actual moral beliefs and norms that influence how individuals behave, while metaethics delves into the language, concepts, and reasoning methods used in normative ethics. "Moral norms" refer to the accepted standards of right and wrong behavior within a given society or community. These norms are essential for establishing a framework of common morality that consists of universally affirmed norms, obligations, and virtues. In contrast to common morality, particular moralities present specific, nonuniversal, and content-rich norms that may vary across different cultural or professional contexts. Professions often adhere to professional moralities, which are reflected in codes of conduct such as the American

Medical Association's Code for Healthcare Professionals. Additionally, health professionals derive moral guidance not only from professional codes, but also from government regulations and public policy, which shape the ethical landscape within the healthcare sector. Various studies and research projects have explored the role of moral norms in influencing human behavior and decision-making. For instance, research has shown that moral norms can be a key determinant of intentions and behaviors, particularly in domains where there is a conflict between moral norms and personal attitudes. Understanding the impact of moral norms on behavior can provide valuable insights into how individuals navigate ethical dilemmas and make decisions that align with societal expectations and values. Overall, moral norms serve as a crucial foundation for ethical conduct and decision-making within social contexts. By examining the sources and influences of moral norms, researchers and practitioners can gain a deeper understanding of how individuals interpret and apply ethical standards in their interactions, professions, and daily lives. The study of moral norms contributes to the broader discourse on ethics and morality, shedding light on the complexities of human behavior and the factors that shape our moral beliefs and actions.

Moral Dilemmas

Moral dilemmas arise when legitimate moral norms conflict, requiring careful consideration and resolution. Principlism, a common ethical framework, involves four clusters of prima facie moral principles: respect for autonomy, nonmaleficence, beneficence, and justice. These principles guide ethical decision-making, with each principle upheld unless outweighed by another. Balancing and specification processes help navigate conflicting moral norms, ensuring ethical decisions are made with good reasons, achievable goals, and minimal negative impact while treating all parties impartially. Given the complexity of applying moral norms in diverse circumstances and the potential for moral disagreement in pluralistic societies, individuals must strive to justify their ethical judgments based on coherent interpretations of common morality. Legitimate moral disagreements are inevitable, but parties should aim to demonstrate the moral coherence and preferability of their ethical positions to foster constructive dialogue and ethical decision-making.

Moral dilemmas are situations in which legitimate moral norms come into conflict, presenting individuals with challenging decisions that require careful consideration and resolution. Principlism, a widely used ethical framework, consists of four clusters of prima facie moral principles: respect for autonomy, nonmaleficence, beneficence, and justice. These principles serve as guiding values in ethical decision-making, with each principle being upheld unless it is outweighed by another principle in a particular context. When faced with conflicting moral norms, individuals often engage in balancing and specification processes to navigate these dilemmas effectively. Balancing involves weighing the importance of each conflicting norm and determining which should take precedence in a given situation. Specification entails clarifying and refining the application of moral principles to ensure that ethical decisions are made with good reasons, achievable goals, and minimal negative consequences, while also treating all parties involved impartially. The application of moral norms in diverse circumstances can be complex, especially in pluralistic societies where different individuals or groups may hold varying ethical beliefs. In such contexts, individuals are encouraged to justify their ethical judgments based on coherent interpretations of common morality, seeking to align their decisions with widely accepted moral principles. While legitimate moral disagreements are inevitable, parties involved in ethical debates should strive to demonstrate the moral coherence and preferability of their ethical positions. By engaging in constructive dialogue and presenting well-reasoned arguments, individuals can work towards resolving moral conflicts and making ethically sound decisions that uphold the principles of common morality. Navigating moral dilemmas involves understanding and applying ethical principles such as respect for autonomy, nonmaleficence, beneficence, and justice. By engaging in balancing and specification processes, individuals can address conflicting moral norms and make decisions that are ethically justifiable and considerate of all parties involved. In pluralistic societies, promoting constructive dialogue and seeking moral coherence can help foster ethical decision-making and resolve disagreements in a manner that upholds shared moral values.

Common Morality and Universal Morality

Common morality refers to a set of universal norms and precepts that are shared by all individuals who are rational and moral (Tate & Clair, 2023). It represents a foundational framework of moral principles that are considered valid by all people committed to morality (English, 2005). This concept suggests that there are fundamental moral duties that emerge from this common morality, forming the basis for ethical decision-making and behavior (Herissone-Kelly, 2022). The common morality is characterized by a set of very general norms that are accepted by anyone committed to the institution of morality (Herissone-Kelly, 2022). It serves as a moral compass that guides individuals in understanding what is right and wrong, just, and fair (Dahl, 2023). This shared moral framework is essential for fostering ethical behavior and promoting the well-being of individuals as well as society as a whole (Goodpaster, 2017). The notion of common morality is rooted in the idea that there are universal moral values and principles that transcend individual beliefs and cultural differences (Susewind & Hoelzl, 2014). It emphasizes the importance of moral values such as justice, fairness, and compassion, which are central to most people's moral self-definitions (Kavussanu & Al-Yaaribi, 2019). This shared understanding of morality helps shape individuals' moral identities and guides their moral decision-making (Kvaran & Sanfey, 2010). In essence, common morality provides a common ground for ethical conduct, emphasizing the importance of moral integrity, respect for others, and the promotion of the common good (Li et al., 2023). It serves as a moral foundation that underpins societal norms, ethical principles, and individual moral behavior, contributing to a more just and harmonious society (Benatar, 2003). By recognizing and adhering to common moral principles, individuals can navigate moral dilemmas, uphold ethical standards, and contribute to a more morally upright and cohesive community (Robins–Browne et al., 2018).

Common morality is based on fundamental principles that guide ethical behavior and decision-making. These principles are derived from a shared understanding of universal moral values and principles that transcend individual beliefs and cultural differences. Zölzer (2016). One of the core tenets of common morality is the emphasis on principles such as justice, fairness, compassion, and respect for others. These principles are essential for promoting the well-being of individuals and society as a whole. Another key aspect of common morality is the belief in universal moral norms accepted by all rational individuals committed to morality. These norms provide a common ground for ethical conduct and help individuals differentiate between right and wrong. The common morality framework consists of a shared set of general norms valid for all individuals committed to morality. Moreover, common morality theory suggests the presence of an informal public moral system involving all individuals, which aids in ethical decision-making (Robertson et al., 2007). This shared moral framework is crucial for resolving disputes, guiding clinical practice, and shaping health policy (Iltis, 2018). Adhering to common moral principles enables individuals to navigate moral dilemmas, uphold ethical standards, and contribute to a just and harmonious society. In essence, common morality revolves around universal moral values, shared ethical principles, and a collective understanding of right and wrong that transcends individual beliefs and cultural differences. By upholding these core tenets, individuals can maintain moral integrity, advance the common good, and foster a more ethical and cohesive community.

Christian Ethics and Common Morality

In the context of bioethics, moral norms in Christian ethics play a significant role in guiding ethical decision-making and shaping moral frameworks. Christian bioethics draws upon foundational principles rooted in Christian teachings and beliefs to address ethical dilemmas in healthcare and biomedical research.

Sanctity of Life

The principle of the sanctity of life emphasizes the inherent value and dignity of every human life, guiding ethical considerations related to issues such as euthanasia, abortion, and end-of-life care. In the realm of Christian ethics and common morality, the principle of the sanctity of life is of paramount importance. This principle underscores the intrinsic value and dignity of every human life, shaping ethical considerations surrounding contentious issues like euthanasia, abortion, and end-of-life care. Rooted in Christian teachings, the concept of the sanctity of life asserts that human life is sacred and warrants protection and reverence at all stages. Christian ethics, underpinned by the sanctity of life principle, highlights the divine essence of human life, recognizing each individual as being made in the image of God (Gielen et al., 2009). This perspective accentuates the inherent worth of every person, irrespective of circumstances, serving as a foundation for ethical decision-making concerning matters of life and death.

The sanctity of life principle is in harmony with common morality, acknowledging the universal value of human life and the moral obligation to safeguard and uphold it (Quaghebeur et al., 2009). This shared moral framework transcends individual convictions and cultural disparities, providing a basis for ethical behavior and decision-making. Within Christian ethics, the sanctity of life principle guides adherents to uphold the dignity and value of every human being, influencing their positions on issues such as euthanasia and abortion. This principle underscores the moral duty to preserve life, foster human well-being, and alleviate suffering, reflecting a commitment to the common good and the welfare of all individuals (Albanesi et al., 2020). Moreover, the sanctity of life principle intersects with the Christian ideals of love and compassion, prompting believers to demonstrate empathy and compassion towards those in vulnerable circumstances, including the terminally ill, the unborn, and the elderly (Madadin et al., 2020). By honoring the sanctity of life, individuals are called to acknowledge the intrinsic worth of every individual, advocate for justice and mercy, and strive to endorse choices and actions that affirm life.

Human Dignity

Christian ethics uphold the concept of human dignity, emphasizing the respect and worth of every individual. This principle informs decisions regarding informed consent, patient autonomy, and the protection of vulnerable populations. In the context of Christian ethics and common morality, the principle of human dignity plays a central role in guiding ethical decision-making and shaping moral conduct. Christian ethics emphasize the inherent worth and respect due to every individual, reflecting the belief that each person is created in the image of God and possesses intrinsic value Stievano et al. (2022). This foundational belief underscores the importance of upholding human dignity in all interactions and decisions, recognizing the sacredness and worth of each individual. The concept of human dignity, deeply rooted in Christian teachings, aligns with common morality by emphasizing the universal value of every human life and the moral imperative to treat individuals with respect and dignity (P, 2020). This shared moral framework transcends cultural boundaries and individual beliefs, providing a common ground for ethical considerations related to informed consent, patient autonomy, and the protection of vulnerable populations. In the context of Christian ethics, the principle of human dignity informs decisions regarding healthcare practices, emphasizing the importance of respecting patients' autonomy, honoring their inherent worth, and upholding their dignity throughout the care process (Shaffer et al., 2022). This ethical framework underscores the moral duty to protect the vulnerable, promote justice, and ensure that individuals are treated with compassion and respect. Moreover, the concept of human dignity intersects with Christian values of love, compassion, and justice, guiding believers to advocate for the well-being and dignity of all individuals, especially those in need or facing challenging circumstances (Ilesanmi, 2023). By upholding human dignity, individuals are called to demonstrate empathy, compassion, and a commitment to promoting the flourishing and dignity of others.

Compassion and Care

The Christian value of compassion and care underscores the importance of empathy, kindness, and holistic care in healthcare settings. This principle guides healthcare providers in providing compassionate and patient-centered care. In the context of Christian ethics and common morality, the concepts of compassion and care hold significant importance in guiding ethical behavior and decision-making. Both compassion and care are deeply intertwined with the principles of respect, empathy, and the recognition of the intrinsic value of every individual. Christian ethics emphasize the practice of compassion and care as essential virtues that reflect the teachings of love, kindness, and empathy found in the Christian tradition (Borgstrom & Walter, 2015). The concept of compassion is rooted in the understanding of suffering and the deep realization of others' pain, leading to a commitment to alleviate that suffering (Ergin et al., 2019). Similarly, care is viewed as a moral imperative that involves nurturing, supporting, and attending to the needs of others with empathy and kindness (Shahzad et al., 2014). In the realm of common morality, compassion and care are regarded as fundamental aspects of ethical conduct that transcend cultural boundaries and individual beliefs (Blomqvist et al., 2022). These concepts underscore the importance of relational ethics, emphasizing care as a relationship rather than a commodity (Blomqvist et al., 2022). Compassion, in particular, is seen as a moral sentiment that drives individuals to prevent and alleviate suffering, promoting a sense of interconnectedness and shared humanity (Ortega-Galán et al., 2021). Within Christian ethics, the practice of compassion and care informs decisions related to healthcare, emphasizing the importance of patient-centered care, empathy, and the protection of vulnerable populations (Smith-MacDonald et al., 2019). These virtues guide healthcare providers to treat patients with dignity, respect their autonomy, and provide compassionate support during times of illness and distress (Yüksel et al., 2022). Moreover, the concepts of compassion and care intersect with Christian values of love, mercy, and justice, prompting individuals to demonstrate empathy, kindness, and a sense of responsibility towards others (Robson, 2022). By embodying these virtues, individuals can foster a culture of compassion, promote ethical behavior, and contribute to the well-being and flourishing of society as a whole.

Justice and Equity

Christian ethics advocate for justice and equity in healthcare, promoting fair treatment, access to care, and advocacy for marginalized populations. This principle informs discussions on healthcare disparities, resource allocation, and social determinants of health. In the realm of Christian ethics and common morality, the principles of justice and equity are foundational pillars that guide ethical decision-making and promote fairness and equality in society. Both justice and equity are closely linked to values such as respect, fairness, and the acknowledgment of the inherent worth of every individual. Christian ethics stresses the significance of justice and equity as crucial elements of moral behavior, reflecting teachings of righteousness, compassion, and social responsibility within the Christian tradition (Dangi & Petrick, (2021). Justice emphasizes the moral duty to uphold fairness, equality, and the rule of law, ensuring just and equitable treatment of individuals (Smith et al., 2018). On the other hand, equity is rooted in the principle of social justice, highlighting the importance of addressing disparities and fostering fairness in the allocation of resources and opportunities (Purificacion et al., 2015). Within common morality, justice and equity are recognized as universal ethical principles that surpass cultural boundaries and individual beliefs, offering a shared framework for advancing equality and fairness (Ndumbe-Eyoh et al., 2021). These concepts underscore the necessity of tackling social inequalities, advocating for the rights of marginalized groups, and striving for a more just and equitable society (Boylan, 2016). In the context of Christian ethics, the principles of justice and equity guide decisions related to social welfare, support for marginalized populations, and the advancement of human rights (Naphan-Kingery et al., 2019). These virtues prompt individuals to combat injustice, champion equality, and endeavor to establish a more just and equitable society for all (Hunt & Godard, 2013). Furthermore, the concepts of justice and equity intersect with Christian values of love, compassion, and solidarity, motivating believers to pursue social change, address systemic injustices, and enhance the well-being of all individuals (McGlothen-Bell et al., 2022). By upholding principles of justice and equity, individuals can contribute to constructing a more just, fair, and inclusive society that respects the dignity and rights of every person.

CHAPTER KEY TERMS

Autonomy - A moral and ethical principle that emphasizes respecting individuals' self-governance and personal decision-making abilities, particularly in healthcare contexts.

Beneficence - An ethical principle that involves actions intended to benefit others, which includes promoting the welfare of individuals and contributing positively to their well-being.

Bioethics - A field of study that deals with the ethical implications of biological and medical procedures and technologies, addressing moral issues in healthcare, life sciences, and biotechnology.

Christian Ethics - Moral principles derived from Christian teachings, which guide ethical decision-making and influence moral behavior, particularly in contexts like healthcare.

Compassion and Care - Fundamental aspects of ethical conduct that involve empathy, kindness, and active efforts to alleviate suffering and provide support.

Common Morality - A set of moral norms that are universally recognized and upheld by all rational, ethical individuals, forming the foundation for ethical decision-making across different contexts.

Descriptive Ethics - The study of people's beliefs about morality, examining the ethical norms that actually guide human behavior in various social contexts.

Dignity, Human - The principle that all individuals possess an inherent worth and should be treated with respect and consideration, a core tenet in many ethical frameworks.

Equity - A principle focused on fairness and justice, particularly in allocating resources or opportunities to ensure equal treatment for all individuals.

Justice - An ethical principle concerned with fairness and the equitable distribution of benefits and burdens, emphasizing the need for moral righteousness in societal practices.

Metaethics - A branch of ethics that analyzes the nature, scope, and meaning of moral judgments and terms, exploring the foundations of ethical theories.

Moral Dilemmas - Situations where conflicting moral principles or norms require careful consideration and decision-making to resolve ethical conflicts.

Moral Norms - Established standards of behavior that are considered right or wrong within a specific community or society, guiding individual and collective actions.

Nonmaleficence - An ethical principle that entails avoiding harm to others, commonly upheld in medical and ethical decision-making to prevent negative outcomes.

Normative Ethics - A branch of ethics that seeks to establish the norms and principles that should guide moral conduct, determining what is morally right or wrong.

Nonnormative Ethics - Ethical theories or perspectives that do not rely on established norms or standards, often exploring alternative approaches to conventional ethical frameworks.

Principlism - An approach in bioethics that uses a set of four prima facie moral principles (autonomy, nonmaleficence, beneficence, and justice) to navigate ethical dilemmas.

Sanctity of Life - A principle emphasizing the inherent value and dignity of all human life, often guiding decisions regarding life and death matters in ethical and religious contexts.

DISCUSSION QUESTIONS

1. **Resource Allocation in a Pandemic**

   Scenario: Imagine a scenario where a hospital has only one ventilator left but two patients need it urgently: an elderly priest and a young father of three. How would the principles of justice and equity guide the decision-making process in this situation? Discuss the ethical implications of choosing one patient over the other.

2. **Genetic Engineering Debate**

   Scenario: A couple wants to use genetic engineering to ensure their child does not inherit a fatal genetic disorder present in their family. Using the principle of sanctity of life, discuss whether it is ethical to modify an embryo to prevent disease. How does this align with or challenge Christian ethics?

3. **Autonomy vs. Beneficence in Mental Health**

   Scenario: A patient diagnosed with severe depression wants to refuse medication, preferring natural remedies, despite medical advice to the contrary. How should the healthcare provider balance respect for the patient's autonomy with the principle of beneficence? What would be the morally appropriate action according to normative ethics?

4. End-of-Life Care Choices

Scenario: An elderly patient with terminal cancer requests physician-assisted suicide to avoid prolonged suffering. Discuss how Christian ethics might interpret the sanctity of life in this context. What moral dilemmas arise when autonomy conflicts with the sanctity of life principle?

5. Informed Consent in a Rural Clinic

Scenario: A doctor in a rural area with limited healthcare access performs life-saving procedures without fully explaining the risks to patients due to time constraints and educational barriers. Is this a violation of human dignity and informed consent? Discuss the ethical challenges faced by healthcare providers in such settings.

6. Healthcare Disparities and Equity

Scenario: In a city, residents of a poor neighborhood have significantly less access to healthcare services than those in wealthier areas. Explore the roles of justice and equity in addressing this disparity. What ethical measures could be implemented to improve fairness in healthcare access?

7. Volunteer Work in Dangerous Regions

Scenario: A volunteer nurse is considering whether to serve in a war-torn region where medical needs are critical but personal risk is high. Discuss how the principles of compassion, care, and nonmaleficence should influence her decision. What moral obligations are at play here?

8. Corporate Responsibility in Healthcare

Scenario: A pharmaceutical company has developed a vaccine for a deadly virus but plans to sell it at a high profit margin, making it unaffordable for many who need it most. Analyze this situation through the lens of common morality and the Christian ethical imperative of justice and equity.

9. **Parental Rights and Child Welfare**

   Scenario: Parents refuse a life-saving blood transfusion for their child based on their religious beliefs. How should healthcare providers respond? Discuss the conflict between parental rights and the ethical duty to protect the child's life and well-being.

10. **AI in Medical Decision-Making**

    Scenario: A hospital uses AI systems to help make treatment decisions. One system recommended a less aggressive treatment for a terminally ill patient, which surprised the care team. Explore how principles of nonmaleficence and beneficence can be applied to the use of artificial intelligence in healthcare. What are the potential benefits and pitfalls of relying on AI for ethical decision-making?

CHAPTER 4

MORAL CHARACTER

In Christian bioethics, moral character refers to the ethical virtues, values, and principles that guide individuals in making moral decisions and conducting themselves ethically in healthcare and biomedical settings. In Christian bioethics, moral character is shaped by foundational Christian teachings, values, and beliefs, influencing how individuals approach ethical dilemmas, interact with patients, and uphold moral standards in healthcare practice. Christian bioethics emphasizes the importance of cultivating moral character traits such as compassion, integrity, honesty, humility, and respect for human dignity. These virtues are integral to ethical decision-making and the provision of compassionate and patient-centered care in healthcare settings. Moral character in Christian bioethics reflects a commitment to upholding ethical principles, respecting the sanctity of life, and promoting the well-being of individuals while adhering to Christian values and teachings. Healthcare professionals who embody strong moral character in Christian bioethics demonstrate a commitment to ethical conduct, integrity, and compassion in their interactions with patients, colleagues, and the broader healthcare community. Upholding moral character traits rooted in Christian ethics fosters trust, respect, and ethical practice in healthcare, ensuring that individuals receive care that aligns with Christian values and principles of compassion, justice, and human dignity. In the context of bioethics, the concept of moral character plays a crucial role in guiding ethical decision-making and professional conduct.

Virtue Ethics

In Christian bioethics, moral character is often viewed through the lens of virtue ethics, which focuses on cultivating virtuous traits and moral excellence in individuals. Virtues such as compassion, integrity, honesty, and empathy are considered essential for healthcare professionals to uphold ethical standards and provide compassionate care to patients.

Virtue ethics, within the realm of bioethics and moral character, is a philosophical approach that focuses on the development of moral character and virtues in individuals. Unlike other ethical theories that emphasize rules, consequences, or duties, virtue ethics places importance on cultivating virtuous traits such as compassion, empathy, honesty, and integrity (Benatar & Upshur, 2014). Virtue ethics is a philosophical approach in bioethics that focuses on cultivating moral character and virtues in individuals. Unlike deontological or consequentialist ethical theories, which prioritize adherence to rules or consideration of outcomes, virtue ethics underscores the significance of developing virtuous traits such as compassion, empathy, honesty, and integrity. This approach, as outlined by Benatar and Upshur (2014), emphasizes the intrinsic value of character traits and the importance of nurturing these qualities in individuals to guide their ethical decision-making processes.

This ethical framework encourages individuals to embody and practice virtues that lead to ethical behavior and decision-making. In the context of bioethics, virtue ethics goes beyond mere adherence to rules or principles, delving into the character of the individual involved in ethical dilemmas. It emphasizes the importance of developing virtuous traits that guide individuals in making morally sound decisions (Benatar & Upshur, 2014). By focusing on the cultivation of virtues such as compassion and empathy, virtue ethics aims to foster a moral character that leads to ethical actions and outcomes in the field of bioethics. In virtue ethics, the focus is not solely on determining what actions are morally right or wrong based on rules or consequences, but rather on fostering a virtuous character that naturally leads individuals to act in morally commendable ways. By prioritizing the cultivation of virtues, individuals are encouraged to embody ethical principles in their daily lives, making ethical decision-making a reflection of their character rather than a strict adherence to external guidelines. In virtue ethics, the emphasis on virtues aligns with the idea that ethical behavior stems from the individual's internal disposition. By developing virtues such as honesty, compassion, and integrity, individuals are better equipped to navigate complex moral dilemmas and make decisions that are not only morally sound but also reflective of their character strengths.

In bioethics, virtue ethics emphasizes the significance of virtues such as empathy and compassion in healthcare settings. These virtues are essential for healthcare providers to effectively care for patients, understand their needs, and make ethical decisions that prioritize the well-being of individuals (Fairchild, 2020). By cultivating virtues like compassion, healthcare professionals can enhance the quality of care they provide and promote ethical practices in the healthcare setting. Moreover, virtue ethics in bioethics encourages individuals to develop a moral character that aligns with ethical principles and values. By focusing on virtues such as compassion, integrity, and respect, individuals can navigate complex ethical issues in healthcare with wisdom and moral discernment (Lebacqz, 2016). This approach emphasizes the importance of character development and the cultivation of virtues that lead to ethical conduct and decision-making in bioethics.

Professional Responsibilities

In Christian bioethics, moral character is closely tied to healthcare providers' professional responsibilities. Being a virtuous physician, nurse, or social worker entails more than just following institutional expectations and standards of practice; it also entails embodying moral virtues that are fundamental to the practice of medicine. Virtue ethics, particularly in the context of professional responsibilities, emphasizes the development of moral character and virtues that guide ethical behavior and decision-making. This ethical framework focuses on cultivating virtues such as compassion, integrity, and honesty to shape the moral character of individuals in professional roles (Oakley & Cocking, 2001). In professions where complexities and constraints create unique moral demands, traits that are considered vices in ordinary life may be praised as virtues within the context of professional roles (Oakley & Cocking, 2001).

Within the field of bioethics, virtue ethics plays a crucial role in addressing disparities and barriers faced by individuals, such as the transgender population, in accessing healthcare services (Wimberly, 2019). By promoting virtues like compassion and competence among healthcare providers, virtue ethics can enhance the quality of care and ensure that individuals receive compassionate and knowledgeable support (Wimberly, 2019). In the context of professional roles, virtue ethics underscores the importance of virtues such as empathy and integrity in guiding ethical conduct and decision-making (Oakley & Cocking, 2001). By focusing on the development of virtuous traits, individuals can navigate ethical dilemmas with wisdom, compassion, and a commitment to upholding ethical standards in their professional practice (Oakley & Cocking, 2001). Moreover, virtue ethics in professional settings encourages individuals to embody virtues that go beyond mere adherence to rules or principles. By cultivating virtues such as honesty, fairness, and respect, professionals can promote a culture of integrity, compassion, and excellence in their respective fields (Doukas, 2003). This approach emphasizes the importance of character development and the cultivation of virtues that lead to ethical conduct and responsible professional practice.

Moral Excellence

In Christian bioethics, moral character is linked to the pursuit of moral excellence and integrity in healthcare practice. Lives of exemplary moral excellence, characterized by virtues such as compassion, integrity, and faithfulness, serve as models for healthcare professionals to aspire to in their ethical conduct.

By focusing on moral character and virtues in the context of Christian bioethics, healthcare professionals can uphold ethical standards, provide compassionate care, and navigate complex ethical dilemmas with integrity and moral excellence. Cultivating moral character traits rooted in Christian values contributes to the ethical practice of healthcare and promotes the well-being of patients and the broader community. Virtue ethics, in the context of moral excellence, focuses on the development of moral character and virtues that lead to ethical behavior and decision-making. It emphasizes the cultivation of virtues such as compassion, integrity, and honesty to promote moral excellence in individuals. Moral excellence, within the framework of virtue ethics, refers to the attainment of virtuous traits and the embodiment of ethical values that contribute to one's moral character and conduct. In professions and fields where moral excellence is paramount, such as bioethics, virtue ethics plays a crucial role in guiding individuals towards ethical practices and moral integrity (Morales-Sánchez & Cabello-Medina, 2015). By emphasizing virtues like compassion, empathy, and honesty, virtue ethics encourages individuals to strive for moral excellence in their professional roles, promoting ethical conduct and responsible decision-making (Morales-Sánchez & Cabello-Medina, 2015). The pursuit of moral excellence through virtue ethics involves the development of character traits that are considered ethically admirable, such as integrity, fairness, and respect (Morales-Sánchez & Cabello-Medina, 2015). Individuals who cultivate these virtues can improve their moral character, exhibit ethical behavior, and contribute to the promotion of moral excellence in their professional responsibilities. Moreover, virtue ethics in the context of moral excellence underscores the importance of integrating virtues into professional roles and responsibilities (Armstrong, 2006). By embodying virtues such as compassion and competence, individuals can strive for excellence in their professional practice, uphold ethical standards, and promote the well-being of those they serve (Armstrong, 2006).

CHAPTER KEY TERMS

Bioethics - The study of ethical and moral implications in medical and biological research. This field addresses the ethical concerns arising from advances in medicine, biotechnology, and related areas.

Compassion - A virtue that involves empathetically sharing and addressing the suffering of others. Essential in healthcare, it motivates practitioners to alleviate patient suffering with sensitivity.

Empathy - The ability to understand and share the feelings of another person. In a healthcare context, empathy is crucial for delivering patient-centered care that acknowledges and respects the patient's emotional and physical experiences.

Human Dignity - A core principle in bioethics that asserts the inherent worth and respect owed to each individual, irrespective of their condition or characteristics.

Integrity - The adherence to strong moral principles, including honesty. In the healthcare sector, integrity is crucial for maintaining ethical standards and trustworthiness in professional conduct.

Moral Character - The ensemble of ethical virtues and traits that define an individual's behavior and decision-making processes. In the context of Christian bioethics, this often aligns with the virtues taught in Christian doctrine.

Sanctity of Life - A concept in Christian ethics that views all human life as sacred and untouchable. This principle influences decisions in healthcare, particularly concerning issues like end-of-life care, abortion, and euthanasia.

Virtue Ethics - A philosophical approach that prioritizes character and virtue over duty or consequence in moral philosophy. It focuses on cultivating personal virtues that encourage ethical behavior.

DISCUSSION QUESTIONS

1. **Resource Allocation**

   Scenario: Imagine a hospital is facing a shortage of life-saving medication. How should a healthcare provider prioritize patients? Discuss how virtues such as compassion, integrity, and respect for human dignity might guide their decisions.

2. **End-of-Life Care**

   Scenario: A patient in severe pain requests euthanasia, but it conflicts with the healthcare provider's Christian ethical views on the sanctity of life. How should the provider handle this request? What virtues are at play, and how might they resolve the ethical dilemma?

3. **Patient Autonomy**

   Scenario: A Christian nurse disagrees with a patient's decision to decline a certain type of treatment due to personal beliefs. How should the nurse balance respect for the patient's autonomy with her own commitment to promoting well-being? Which virtues could guide her actions?

4. **Cultural Sensitivity**

   Scenario: A healthcare team is treating a patient from a different cultural background that has distinct beliefs about healthcare. Discuss how virtues like empathy and humility could assist the team in providing culturally sensitive care.

5. **Truth-Telling**

   Scenario: A doctor knows that disclosing a full diagnosis will likely cause severe emotional distress to the patient. Should the doctor withhold part of the information? Examine this dilemma through the virtues of honesty and compassion.

6. **Professional Boundaries**

   Scenario: A social worker feels a personal connection with a client that could potentially interfere with professional judgment. What virtues should guide the social worker in maintaining professional boundaries while being compassionate and empathetic?

7. **Pediatric Care**

   Scenario: Parents of a pediatric patient refuse a procedure that medical professionals believe is necessary for the child's health. How should healthcare providers approach this situation while respecting family autonomy and ensuring the child's well-being? Which Christian virtues might influence their approach?

8. **Healthcare Equity**

   Scenario: A medical administrator notices that certain demographics in the community are underserved. Discuss how virtues such as justice and fairness can guide efforts to improve access to healthcare for these populations.

9. **Whistleblowing**

   Scenario: A nurse discovers unethical practices at her healthcare facility. Discuss the moral conflict of whistleblowing through the lens of virtues like courage, integrity, and loyalty. What steps should the nurse take according to virtue ethics?

10. **Confidentiality**

   Scenario: A healthcare professional is pressured by family members to reveal confidential information about a patient's condition. How should the professional handle this pressure? Discuss the virtues that might

CHAPTER 5

MORAL STATUS

I n bioethics, various theories exist to determine the moral status of entities such as humans, animals, and even chimeric beings. One prevalent theory is rooted in Western moral philosophy, emphasizing rational, logical, and objective approaches to addressing complex moral issues (Bowman, 2004). This theory often relies on principles like beneficence, autonomy, and justice to guide ethical decision-making (Chukwuneke et al., 2014). However, the application of these principles can vary significantly across cultures, as seen in Africa, where cultural influences shape the understanding and application of bioethical principles (Chukwuneke et al., 2014). Furthermore, the moral status of entities, particularly in the context of research involving chimeric animals, remains a topic of ethical debate within the bioethics community (Marshall et al., 2022). The concept of moral status is critical in determining how these entities should be treated, as well as the ethical considerations that must be taken into account.

Additionally, the role of empathy and moral sensitivity among healthcare professionals, including physicians, plays a significant role in shaping bioethical decision-making (Alyousefi et al., 2021). Empathy and moral sensitivity are crucial components in healthcare within the realm of bioethics, particularly concerning the assessment of moral status. Empathy allows healthcare professionals to understand the emotions and experiences of patients, fostering a deeper connection and enabling them to make decisions that benefit the patient (Galdames et al., 2020). This emotional intelligence is essential in navigating complex ethical dilemmas and ensuring that decisions prioritize the well-being of individuals. Moreover, moral sensitivity plays a significant role in enhancing the understanding of moral issues. It is emphasized that empathy is a key factor in improving moral sensitivity, which in turn aids in making ethically sound decisions (Rezapour-Mirsaleh et al., 2021). This aligns with the argument that moral sensitivity can be heightened by enhancing empathy, a personal factor, and by fostering an ethical climate within healthcare organizations (Jo & Kim, 2017). In bioethics, the concept of human dignity is closely related to moral status. Human dignity underscores the inherent worth and value of human life, guiding ethical decision-making processes and ensuring that individuals are treated with respect and fairness (Baertschi, 2014). This notion of dignity is intertwined with empathy and moral sensitivity, as it calls for a deep understanding and consideration of the moral significance of individuals in healthcare settings.

Furthermore, feminist perspectives in bioethics challenge traditional approaches by highlighting the importance of considering concrete cases and the moral significance of various groups, such as marginalized communities (Drezgić, 2012). Feminist bioethics focuses on addressing the oppression of women within healthcare systems, critiquing standard bioethical principles, and advocating for a more diverse and inclusive ethical reflection community (Giblin, 1997). It also calls for a reevaluation of liberal individualism in mainstream bioethics and encourages a critical examination of the discipline's social location and loyalties (Giblin, 1997). By highlighting the concrete forms of oppression faced by women in healthcare settings, feminist bioethics aims to promote a more just and equitable healthcare system that considers the diverse needs and experiences of all individuals (Giblin, 1997). This critique underscores the need for a more inclusive and socially aware approach to bioethical issues. Additionally, the concept of human dignity is central to many bioethical discussions, emphasizing the inherent worth and value of human life (Baertschi, 2014).

Sentience

In bioethical considerations, the moral status of entities, particularly in the context of sentience, plays a crucial role. Sentience, the capacity to experience feelings and sensations, is often regarded as a significant factor in determining moral status (Martin, 2019). While vulnerability and sentience are distinct concepts, with sentience being a sufficient reason to ascribe moral status to a being, vulnerability draws attention to those who may be more likely to be denied what they are due (Martin, 2019). This distinction underscores the complexity of ethical considerations when evaluating the moral status of different entities. In the realm of bioethics, the possession of sentience is considered a necessary and sufficient condition for moral status, as it implies having an interest in furthering one's welfare (Lederman, 2022). The debate surrounding the moral significance of sentience extends to various entities, including animals and even chimeric beings involved in research (Koplin, 2019). The consideration of sentience in bioethical discussions is essential for addressing ethical dilemmas and ensuring the well-being of sentient beings (Browning & Veit, 2023). Moreover, the acknowledgment of animal sentience is fundamental not only to animal welfare but also to various disciplines, highlighting the interconnectedness of ethical considerations and scientific understanding (Demin et al., 2018). The recognition of sentience in animals, including fish, raises important questions about their emotional lives, pain perception, and welfare (Bekoff, 2007). This awareness prompts a reevaluation of practices such as factory farming, emphasizing the ethical implications of disregarding the sentience of animals (Cockshaw, 2021).

In the context of bioethics, the consideration of sentience is crucial in determining the moral status and ethical treatment of animals. For instance, in a case study involving the use of animals in scientific research, the concept of sentience becomes central to ethical decision-making.

Researchers and ethicists must grapple with the ethical implications of potentially causing pain and suffering to sentient beings during experiments. Imagine a scenario where a research team is conducting a study that involves testing the effects of a new drug on laboratory mice. In this case, the ethical dilemma arises from the awareness that mice are sentient beings capable of experiencing pain and distress. The researchers must carefully consider the welfare of the animals, taking into account their capacity for sentience and the ethical responsibilities that come with it. Recognizing the sentience of the laboratory mice and their ability to suffer, the research team is compelled to implement measures to minimize harm, ensure humane treatment, and prioritize animal welfare throughout the study. This ethical consideration of sentience guides the researchers in making decisions that align with principles of compassion, respect, and ethical conduct in animal research. This case study exemplifies how the concept of sentience in bioethics serves as a critical ethical framework for addressing the moral implications of using sentient beings in scientific experiments. By integrating considerations of sentience into decision-making processes, researchers can uphold ethical standards and promote the well-being of animals involved in research activities.

Theories of Sentience

There are various theories that determine a being's sentience. Biological naturalism argues that sentience originates from biological processes in the brain. Conscious mental states are caused by microphysical processes in the brain and are emergent properties of the brain's higher-level functions. Functionalism suggests that mental states, including sentience, are defined by their functional roles rather than their physical properties. The phenomenonal consciousness theory focuses on the qualitative aspects of conscious experience, emphasizing subjective experiences that are not accessible through objective measures. Panpsychism posits that consciousness is a fundamental feature of the physical world, extending sentience to all elements of the universe. Integrated information theory proposes that consciousness arises from the integration of information in a network. Emergentism argues that sentience is a novel property of complex systems that cannot be predicted based on the properties of individual components. Cognitive theories of consciousness link sentience to cognitive processes and functions, suggesting that the ability to perform higher-level cognitive tasks indicates sentience. Behaviorism infers sentience from observable behaviors rather than subjective experiences.

Biological Naturalism

Developed by John Searle, this perspective argues that sentience arises from certain biological processes, specifically those of the brain. According to biological naturalism, conscious mental states are entirely caused by lower-level microphysical processes in the brain and are themselves higher-level features of the brain. Biological naturalism, as proposed by John Searle, posits that consciousness and sentience are products of specific biological processes, particularly those occurring within the brain. This perspective asserts that conscious mental states are wholly determined by the underlying microphysical activities in the brain and are essentially emergent properties of the brain's higher-level functions. Searle's theory of biological naturalism stands in contrast to other philosophical perspectives on consciousness, such as dualism and functionalism. Dualism, for instance, suggests a separation between the mind and the body, positing that consciousness is a non-physical entity distinct from the physical brain. Functionalism, on the other hand, focuses on the functional role of mental states rather than their specific biological origins.

Functionalism

This theory posits that mental states, including sentience, are constituted solely by their functional role — that is, by their causal relations to sensory inputs, behavioral outputs, and other mental states. A being is sentient if it has functional states that are comparable to human sensory experiences. Functionalism is a prominent theory in the philosophy of mind that suggests mental states, including consciousness and sentience, are defined by their functional roles rather than their specific physical properties. According to functionalism, what makes a mental state what it is is its role or function within the overall system of mental states, sensory inputs, and behavioral outputs. In the context of sentience, functionalism posits that a being is considered sentient if it exhibits functional states that are analogous to human sensory experiences. This means that the capacity for sentience is not dependent on the specific physical makeup of an organism but rather on the functional organization of its mental states and their interactions with the external environment. Functionalism emphasizes the dynamic relationships between mental states and their causal connections to sensory inputs, behavioral responses, and other mental states. This perspective allows for the possibility of different physical systems, such as artificial intelligence or non-human organisms, to exhibit sentience as long as they fulfill the functional criteria for having conscious experiences.

Phenomenal Consciousness Theory (Qualia)

This approach focuses on the qualitative aspects of conscious experience, often referred to as "qualia." Philosophers like David Chalmers emphasize that sentience involves having subjective experiences that are not accessible through objective measures but are felt internally by the individual. The Phenomenal Consciousness Theory, also known as the Qualia Theory, focuses on the qualitative aspects of conscious experiences, often referred to as "qualia." This perspective, championed by philosophers like David Chalmers, highlights that sentience involves subjective experiences that are internally felt by individuals and are not accessible through objective measures. Chalmers and proponents of this theory argue that conscious experiences encompass more than just the external observable behaviors or neural processes; they emphasize the intrinsic, subjective nature of consciousness. Qualia are the raw feelings of experiences, such as the redness of red or the pain of a headache, which cannot be fully captured or explained solely through physical or functional descriptions. Recent research and theoretical models have attempted to establish a connection between subjective conscious experiences and measurable neuronal activity. Studies have explored the neural computations underlying phenomenal consciousness, aiming to understand how specific brain processes give rise to subjective experiences. Additionally, integrated information theory has been proposed to determine the quality and quantity of conscious experiences based on consciousness's physical substrate.

Panpsychism

Panpsychism suggests that sentience, or consciousness, is a fundamental and ubiquitous feature of the physical world. This theory extends the attribute of sentience to all elements of the universe, suggesting that even elementary particles exhibit rudimentary forms of consciousness. Panpsychism is a philosophical theory that posits consciousness as an intrinsic and pervasive aspect of the physical world. According to panpsychism, sentience is not exclusive to complex organisms like humans or animals but is a fundamental property that permeates all levels of existence, including inanimate objects and elementary particles. This perspective suggests that consciousness is not solely generated by complex neural processes but is a fundamental feature of the universe itself. One of the key proponents of panpsychism is the philosopher Alfred North Whitehead, who proposed a process philosophy that views consciousness as a fundamental component of reality. Whitehead's concept of "prehension" suggests that all entities, from the smallest particles to the most complex organisms, possess some form of experiential capacity. Another influential figure in the realm of panpsychism is David Chalmers, who has explored the idea of panexperientialism, which suggests that even basic physical entities have some form of subjective experience. Chalmers argues that consciousness is a fundamental aspect of the universe and cannot be reduced to purely physical or functional processes. Panpsychism challenges traditional views of consciousness and raises profound questions about the nature of reality and the relationship between mind and matter. While this theory may seem radical, it offers a unique perspective on the nature of consciousness and the interconnectedness of all things in the universe.

Integrated Information Theory (IIT)

Proposed by Giulio Tononi, this theory posits that consciousness (and by extension, sentience) arises from the integration of information in a network. According to IIT, a system's consciousness is determined by how efficiently it integrates information, not just the amount of information it processes. Unlike traditional views that focus on the quantity of information processed, IIT emphasizes the quality and efficiency of information integration as the key determinant of consciousness. According to IIT, a system's level of consciousness is directly related to its ability to integrate information in a complex and interconnected manner. This theory suggests that consciousness arises from the interactions and interdependencies among the elements within a system rather than from the individual components themselves. In essence, a system's degree of consciousness is determined by how effectively information is integrated across its network. Tononi's IIT has gained attention in the fields of neuroscience and philosophy of mind for its novel approach to understanding consciousness. By focusing on the dynamic patterns of information flow and integration within neural networks, IIT offers a framework for investigating how subjective experiences emerge from the complex interactions of neural processes.

Emergentism

Emergentism argues that sentience is a new property of complex systems that is not predictable from the properties of the individual components. This approach is often used to describe how consciousness emerges from the complexity of the brain's neural network. Emergentism is a philosophical perspective that argues that sentience or consciousness arises as a new property of complex systems that cannot be predicted from the properties of the individual components. This theory is often used to describe how consciousness emerges from the intricate interactions within the brain's neural network. Emergentism posits that higher-level phenomena, such as consciousness, possess properties that are independent of and not reducible to their lower-level components. The theory suggests that as complex systems, like the brain, organize and interact, new emergent properties, such as consciousness, manifest. This view challenges reductionist approaches that seek to explain complex phenomena solely based on the properties of their constituent parts. Giulio Tononi's Integrated Information Theory (IIT) aligns with emergentism by emphasizing the importance of how information is integrated within a system to determine its level of consciousness. IIT focuses on the emergent nature of consciousness, highlighting that consciousness arises from the dynamic interactions and integration of information within neural networks.

Cognitive Theories of Consciousness

These theories assert that sentience is closely tied to cognitive processes and functions. They argue that a being's capacity to perform certain higher-level cognitive tasks is indicative of its sentience. Cognitive theories of consciousness propose that sentience is intricately linked to cognitive processes and functions. These theories suggest that an entity's ability to engage in higher-level cognitive tasks serves as an indicator of its level of sentience. The capacity to perform complex cognitive functions is seen as a key characteristic of conscious beings. Giulio Tononi's Integrated Information Theory (IIT) aligns with cognitive theories of consciousness by emphasizing the role of information integration in determining the level of consciousness. IIT posits that consciousness emerges from the efficient integration of information within a network, highlighting the cognitive aspect of conscious experiences. Furthermore, cognitive theories of consciousness challenge traditional views that focus solely on the physical or functional aspects of consciousness. These theories underscore the importance of cognitive abilities, such as problem-solving, memory, and decision-making, in understanding the nature of sentience. In the context of animal sentience, cognitive theories play a crucial role in assessing the cognitive capacities of different species and understanding the implications for their welfare and ethical considerations. By examining animals' cognitive abilities, researchers can gain insights into the level of consciousness and sentience present in various species. Overall, cognitive theories of consciousness provide a framework for exploring the relationship between cognitive functions and sentience, shedding light on the cognitive processes that underlie conscious experiences in both humans and other sentient beings.

Behaviorism and Sentience

From a strictly behaviorist perspective, sentience is inferred from the behavior rather than any subjective experience. Although behaviorism itself does not directly address the inner experiences, it defines sentience by observable responses to stimuli. Behaviorism, as a theoretical perspective, focuses on observable behaviors as the primary indicators of sentience rather than delving into subjective experiences. From a behaviorist standpoint, sentience is inferred from an entity's responses to stimuli and its observable actions. This approach does not directly address inner experiences but defines sentience based on external behaviors and reactions. This perspective contrasts with theories that emphasize subjective experiences or cognitive processes as central to understanding sentience. Behaviorism's emphasis on outward behaviors as the basis for inferring sentience aligns with its core tenet of focusing on observable and measurable phenomena. In the context of animal behavior and sentience, behaviorism plays a significant role in studying and interpreting the responses of animals to various stimuli. By observing and analyzing animal behaviors, researchers can make inferences about the presence of sentience and cognitive processes in non-human species. Overall, behaviorism provides a framework for assessing sentience based on external manifestations and responses, highlighting the importance of observable behaviors in understanding the nature of consciousness in both humans and animals.

Rationality

The moral status of entities in bioethics is often intertwined with rational theories that emphasize the importance of rationality, autonomy, and decision-making capacity in determining moral worth. Rationalist conceptions of morality, popular in bioethics, operate by applying a set of rules from a given set of starting conditions to calculate a moral outcome (Lam, (2022). This approach highlights the significance of rational decision-making processes in ethical considerations. In bioethical discussions, the concept of moral status is closely linked to the rational capacity of individuals, particularly in cases where autonomy and decision-making abilities are central to determining moral worth (Subramani & Biller-Andorno, 2022). While Kantian bioethics traditionally upholds unconditional respect for persons based on their rationality, contemporary debates often focus on the concepts of autonomy, emphasizing decision-making capacity and agency (Subramani & Biller-Andorno, 2022). However, it is recognized that rationality and decision-making abilities alone may not be sufficient to fully engage with the concept of respect for persons, especially in healthcare settings (Subramani & Biller-Andorno, 2022). Moreover, the relationship between rationality and moral status extends to various bioethical dilemmas, such as those involving human enhancement, disability, and the treatment of animals (Stramondo, 2016). The consideration of rational capacities and moral psychology is crucial in understanding the diverse perspectives and lived experiences that shape ethical decision-making processes (Stramondo, 2016). Additionally, the acknowledgment of residual cognitive capacities in patients with cognitive motor dissociation raises questions about their moral status and the implications for their well-being (Graham, 2021).

In a case study involving the allocation of scarce medical resources during a public health crisis, rationality plays a crucial role in bioethical decision-making. Imagine a scenario where a hospital is overwhelmed with COVID-19 patients and there is a shortage of ventilators. Healthcare professionals are faced with the ethical dilemma of deciding which patients should receive access to ventilator support based on available medical criteria. In this case, rationality in bioethics involves applying ethical principles, medical evidence, and guidelines to make decisions that maximize the benefits for the greatest number of patients. When allocating ventilators, healthcare providers must take into account factors such as illness severity, prognosis, likelihood of recovery, and potential for long-term quality of life. By employing rational decision-making processes, healthcare professionals can navigate the complex ethical challenges posed by resource scarcity and prioritize patient care based on objective criteria rather than subjective preferences. Rationality in this context helps ensure fairness, transparency, and consistency in decision-making, ultimately promoting the ethical delivery of healthcare services in challenging circumstances.

Moral Agency

Moral agency in bioethics refers to the capacity of individuals to act intentionally and make moral decisions based on their values, beliefs, and understanding of right and wrong. It encompasses the ability to deliberate, choose, and take responsibility for one's actions within the context of ethical considerations (Skalko & Cherry, 2016). Bioethics, as a field of philosophical inquiry, is concerned with examining and advancing arguments about what actions are morally right or wrong, emphasizing the importance of moral agency in ethical decision-making processes (Skalko & Cherry, 2016). The concept of moral agency is closely linked to autonomy, voluntariness, and moral responsibility in bioethical discussions (Skalko & Cherry, 2016). It challenges common assumptions regarding the voluntariness of human actions and underscores the significance of individuals' ability to make informed choices and decisions that align with their values and beliefs (Skalko & Cherry, 2016). Moreover, moral agency plays a crucial role in shaping ethical frameworks and guiding principles in bioethics, emphasizing the importance of individual autonomy and the capacity to act in accordance with one's moral convictions. In the context of bioethical dilemmas, the notion of moral agency highlights the ethical implications of individual actions and decisions for oneself and others (Skalko & Cherry, 2016). It underscores the responsibility individuals have in making choices that consider the well-being and rights of all involved parties, reflecting a commitment to ethical conduct and moral integrity in healthcare and research settings.

An example of moral agency in bioethics can be illustrated by a patient with a terminal illness who is faced with the decision of whether to pursue aggressive treatment or opt for palliative care. In this scenario, the patient's moral agency comes into play as they deliberate on the available options, considering their values, beliefs, and personal goals in the context of their medical condition. The patient's ability to make an informed decision based on their understanding of the treatment options, potential outcomes, and quality of life considerations demonstrates their moral agency. By actively engaging in the decision-making process and taking responsibility for the choice they make, the patient exercises their autonomy and moral responsibility in determining the course of their medical care. Furthermore, healthcare professionals and caregivers play a crucial role in supporting the patient's moral agency by providing clear information, guidance, and emotional support throughout the decision-making process. Respecting the patient's autonomy and empowering them to make choices that align with their values and preferences is essential to upholding their moral agency in healthcare decision-making.

CHAPTER KEY TERMS

Autonomy - The right of competent adults to make informed decisions about their own medical care without coercion.

Beneficence - A principle in ethics that involves the duty to promote good and act in the best interest of others.

Chimeric Beings - Organisms composed of cells from two or more different species; in bioethics, these beings pose special challenges in terms of their moral status and rights.

Empathy - The ability to understand and share the feelings of another, which is critical in healthcare for providing compassionate and sensitive patient care.

Feminist Bioethics - An approach to bioethics that emphasizes understanding and addressing the particular experiences and health needs of women, and advocates for the ethical inclusion of women's perspectives in health care and research.

Human Dignity - A fundamental concept that recognizes the intrinsic worth of all individuals, guiding ethical decision-making and ensuring that individuals are treated with respect and fairness.

Justice - In ethics, particularly bioethics, justice involves the fair distribution of benefits and risks, ensuring that everyone has equal access to the benefits of research and healthcare.

Moral Sensitivity - The ability to detect moral aspects of a situation and how one's actions affect others, which is essential for ethical decision-making in healthcare.

Moral Status - The status granted to an entity that warrants moral consideration or possesses inherent moral rights, often based on characteristics like rationality, sentience, or being part of a certain biological category.

Sentience - The capacity to experience feelings and sensations, considered a critical factor in determining the moral status of animals and other beings.

Vulnerability - Refers to the susceptibility of individuals or groups to harm, often used in ethical discussions about the protection needed by such groups.

DISCUSSION QUESTIONS

1. **Scenario on Autonomy and Ethics:** Imagine a patient who refuses life-saving treatment due to personal beliefs. How should healthcare providers balance respecting the patient's autonomy

with the ethical duty to save lives? What factors should influence their decision?

2. **Biological Naturalism in AI**: Consider a future where artificial intelligence (AI) systems are developed with biological components that might grant them sentience, according to Biological Naturalism. Should these AIs be granted moral status, and if so, what rights should they have?

3. **Empathy in Crisis Situations**: A hospital is overwhelmed during a pandemic, and resources are scarce. How might empathy influence the decisions made by healthcare workers when rationing care? Could too much empathy be detrimental in such situations?

4. **Panpsychism and Environmental Ethics**: If Panpsychism is true, and all matter has some level of consciousness, what are the implications for environmental ethics? How should this influence our interactions with non-living nature?

5. **Feminist Bioethics and Clinical Trials**: A pharmaceutical company has historically excluded pregnant women from clinical trials to avoid potential risks. From a feminist bioethical perspective, discuss the pros and cons of this policy. What changes, if any, should be made?

6. **Human Dignity in End-of-Life Care**: An elderly patient with a terminal illness opts for euthanasia to avoid prolonged suffering, invoking their human dignity. Discuss the ethical complexities this decision presents for the patient's family and healthcare providers.

7. **Justice and Global Health**: A vaccine for a deadly virus is available, but its distribution is uneven globally. How should the principle of justice guide the distribution of this vaccine between countries with different levels of wealth and healthcare infrastructure?

8. **Sentience and Animal Rights**: A new law proposes that any animal proven to have sentience must be granted certain legal protections. Consider a research facility that uses mice in neurological studies. How might this law affect their research practices?

9. **Emergentism and Robot Rights**: In a world where robots exhibit complex behaviors that suggest consciousness, according to Emergentism, should they be treated as moral agents? Discuss the potential societal impacts of recognizing robots as entities with moral status.

10. **Moral Agency in Autonomous Vehicles**: An autonomous vehicle must choose between colliding with a pedestrian or endangering its passengers. Discuss the role of moral agency in programming autonomous vehicles, considering the principles of bioethics like autonomy, justice, and beneficence.

CHAPTER 6

AUTONOMY

I n the field of bioethics, the principle of autonomy is a foundational concept that upholds the right of individuals to make informed decisions about their own health care. Autonomy is a fundamental principle in bioethics, ensuring individuals have the right to make informed decisions about their health care. It is based on the principle of respect for persons, which acknowledges the dignity of individuals and their right to make choices. Informed consent is a crucial application of autonomy, requiring patients to receive full disclosure about their medical conditions, understand the information, and give their consent without coercion. This process ensures patients are aware of potential risks and benefits, can make decisions that align with their values and preferences, and have the capacity to make decisions. Informed consent is a cornerstone of ethical medical practice, protecting patients' rights, promoting transparency, and fostering trust between patients and healthcare professionals.

Mental health treatment, particularly involuntary treatment, raises significant ethical concerns. Mental health professionals often face challenges in making decisions without patient consent, particularly when using psychoactive drugs for various disorders. The ethical dilemmas involve balancing the patient's best interests with autonomy and self-determination. Involuntary psychiatric treatment can lead to debates about coercion and stigmatization. Psychiatric nurses play a crucial role in involuntary treatment, recognizing the importance of respecting patient autonomy. Two case studies illustrate the ethical complexities of managing patients under involuntary psychiatric treatment. Involuntary psychiatric hospitalization presents significant ethical and clinical challenges, necessitating a careful balance between individual rights and the duty to provide necessary care. Mental health professionals, including psychiatrists, grapple with the complexities of decision-making in involuntary treatment scenarios.

Respect for Persons

The Respect of Person standard acknowledges each individual's right to make choices and act on those choices. It is rooted in the belief that all individuals have intrinsic worth and should be treated with dignity. Respect for persons is a fundamental principle in bioethics that emphasizes the importance of recognizing and upholding the autonomy of individuals. Autonomy refers to the ability of individuals to make their own decisions and act in accordance with their own values and beliefs. The principle of respect for persons requires that individuals are treated with dignity and that their right to make choices is acknowledged and respected. This principle is rooted in the belief that all individuals have intrinsic worth and should be afforded the opportunity to exercise their autonomy. It is essential in the field of bioethics because it serves as a guiding principle that ensures that individuals are not only protected from harm but also empowered to make decisions about their own lives and bodies. Respect for persons is often applied in various ethical dilemmas in healthcare, research, and other areas where decisions impact individuals' well-being. For example, in medical decision-making, healthcare providers are expected to respect patients' autonomy by providing them with relevant information about their condition and treatment options and by involving them in the decision-making process. In research ethics, respect for people is reflected in the requirement for informed consent, where individuals are provided with information about the research study and have the opportunity to voluntarily agree to participate based on their understanding of the risks and benefits involved. Overall, respect for persons is a foundational principle in bioethics that underscores the importance of recognizing and honoring individuals' autonomy, dignity, and worth in all ethical considerations and decision-making processes.

Informed Consent

Informed consent, a critical application of autonomy, requires that patients receive full disclosure about their medical conditions and proposed treatments, understand this information, and freely give their consent without coercion. This process ensures that individuals are aware of potential risks and benefits and can make decisions that align with their values and preferences. Informed consent is a critical component of medical ethics that is closely tied to the principle of autonomy. It is a process through which healthcare providers communicate relevant information to patients about their medical condition, proposed treatments, risks, benefits, and alternatives, allowing patients to make informed decisions about their care. The concept of informed consent emphasizes the importance of respecting patients' autonomy by ensuring that they have the necessary information to make decisions that align with their values and preferences.

The process of obtaining informed consent typically involves several key elements. The first is a disclosure. With disclosure, healthcare providers are required to provide patients with clear and comprehensive information about their diagnosis, treatment options, potential risks and benefits, and any available alternatives. This information should be presented in a way that is easily understood by the patient. Privacy and confidentiality form part of respecting a patient's autonomy, which suggests respecting their privacy and keeping their medical information confidential unless consent has been given to share it.

Secondly, there must be understanding. Patients must demonstrate that they have understood the information provided to them. This may involve asking questions, seeking clarification, or discussing the information with their healthcare provider or other trusted individuals.

Furthermore, there must be voluntariness. Patients must be free to make their own decisions without any form of coercion or undue influence. They should not feel pressured or manipulated into consenting to a particular treatment or procedure. Voluntariness is part of autonomy. Autonomy involves decisions made voluntarily, free of any undue influence or coercion. Individuals should have the ability to make health care decisions based on their own values and beliefs rather than being compelled by others.

Finally, there must be capacity. Patients must have the capacity to make decisions about their care. This includes the ability to understand the information provided, appreciate the implications of their decisions, and communicate their choices effectively. Capacity for decision-making includes autonomy, which presumes that individuals have the mental capacity to make their own decisions. This includes being able to understand and weigh the benefits and risks of different treatment options. When individuals are incapable of making decisions (due to age, illness, or mental incapacity), surrogates may be designated to make decisions that align with the individual's preferences and best interests.

Informed consent is a cornerstone of ethical medical practice, essential for upholding patients' rights and promoting shared decision-making between patients and healthcare providers. It serves to protect patients' autonomy, promote transparency in healthcare decision-making, and foster trust between patients and healthcare professionals.

Mental Health Treatment and Ethics

In the realm of mental health treatment, the use of psychiatric treatment, especially in cases of involuntary treatment, raises significant ethical considerations. Mental health professionals often find themselves in challenging situations where they must make decisions about administering treatments without the explicit consent of the patient (Valenti et al., 2013). The practice of involuntary treatment, including the use of psychoactive drugs, is a controversial and widely debated topic that brings to light fundamental ethical questions regarding individual rights and needs

(Clausen et al., 2018). Different categories of drugs can be used for different needs. Antidepressants are used for depression, anxiety disorders, and mood disorders; antipsychotic medications are used for schizophrenia and psychotic disorders; benzodiazepines are used for anxiety disorders; and mood stabilizers are used for bipolar disorders as well as manic and depressive episodes (Baradaran et al., 2020; Shafiekhani & Mirjalili, 2018). The ethical dilemmas surrounding involuntary psychiatric treatment are further complicated by the need to balance the best interests of the patient with considerations of autonomy and self-determination (Dobrin et al., 2019).

Involuntary psychiatric treatment can lead to serious ethical debates, particularly concerning coercion and stigmatization within psychiatric care (Nechita et al., 2020). The literature on compulsory treatment in psychiatric emergencies is limited, highlighting the need for further exploration of the legal, ethical, and practical aspects of such interventions (Becker & Forman, 2020). Additionally, the low adherence to treatment for chronic medical illnesses in the general population adds complexity to the ethical considerations surrounding compulsory treatment in psychiatric settings (Joury et al., 2023). Different ethical concerns regarding psychiatry include paternalism, discussions of stigma and self-contempt, coercion (autonomy), and informed consent (Joury et al., 2023; Rüsch et al., 2013; Sjöstrand et al., 2015; Wynn, 2006).

Autonomy and the Mental Health Practitioner

Psychiatric nurses play a crucial role in involuntary treatment and must be mindful of the ethical implications of promoting compliance, recognizing the importance of respecting patient autonomy even in involuntary treatment scenarios (Vuckovich, 2010). The duty to protect patients undergoing involuntary psychiatric treatment is emphasized, underscoring the medical community's responsibility to safeguard the well-being of individuals whose autonomy has been temporarily overridden (Conrad et al., 2020).

Examples of autonomy that come into conflict with the medical community's care are seen in the following two case study examples:

Case Example 1:

In a psychiatric hospital, a patient with severe schizophrenia is admitted involuntarily due to the risk of harm to themselves and others. The psychiatric nurse assigned to the patient's care acknowledges the ethical implications of encouraging compliance while respecting the patient's autonomy. Despite the involuntary nature of the treatment, the nurse engages in open communication with the patient, explaining the reasons for their hospitalization and involving them in their care decisions to the extent possible. By upholding the patient's autonomy and involving them in the treatment process, the nurse demonstrates a commitment to ethical practice in involuntary psychiatric treatment.

Case Example 2:

A young adult with a history of suicidal ideation is brought to the emergency department under an involuntary psychiatric hold. The psychiatric nurse responsible for the patient's care understands the importance of safeguarding the patient's well-being while respecting their autonomy. The nurse collaborates with the treatment team to develop a care plan that addresses the patient's immediate safety concerns while also considering their preferences and values. Throughout the patient's hospitalization, the nurse advocates for the patient's rights, ensures their dignity is maintained, and provides support to help them navigate the challenges of involuntary treatment.

The two case studies illustrate the ethical complexities and responsibilities of psychiatric nurses when managing patients under involuntary psychiatric treatment. In the first case, a patient with severe schizophrenia is involuntarily admitted to a psychiatric hospital due to potential harm to themselves and others. The assigned nurse navigates the ethical challenge of balancing the need for compliance with treatment while respecting the patient's autonomy. Through open communication and the involvement of the patient in care decisions as much as possible, the nurse upholds the patient's autonomy and demonstrates a commitment to ethical practice in involuntary treatment situations.

The second case involves a young adult with a history of suicidal ideation, admitted under an involuntary psychiatric hold. The nurse prioritizes the patient's well-being and autonomy, collaborating with the treatment team to develop a care plan that considers the patient's safety, preferences, and values. The nurse advocates for the patient's rights, maintains their dignity, and provides support throughout their hospitalization, emphasizing the importance of ethical care and patient advocacy in the context of involuntary psychiatric treatment.

Involuntary Psychiatric Hospitalization and Autonomy

Involuntary psychiatric hospitalization presents significant ethical and clinical challenges, necessitating a careful balance between the rights of the individual and the duty to provide necessary care (Tarsitani et al., 2021). Mental health professionals, including psychiatrists, are at the forefront of these ethical deliberations, grappling with the complexities of decision-making in involuntary treatment scenarios (Sjöstrand et al., 2015). The attitudes and ethical beliefs of psychiatrists regarding compulsory treatment vary, highlighting the need for a deeper understanding of the ethical considerations at play (Kullgren et al., 1996).

CHAPTER KEY TERMS

Autonomy - The right of individuals to make informed, uncoerced decisions about their own healthcare.

Benzodiazepines - A class of psychoactive drugs used to treat anxiety disorders, often discussed in the context of psychiatric ethics and consent.

Capacity - The ability of a patient to understand information relevant to their treatment, appreciate the consequences of decisions, and communicate choices effectively.

Coercion - The practice of compelling an individual to act in a certain way by use of force or threats, at odds with the principle of autonomy in healthcare settings.

Consent, Informed - A process that ensures patients understand their health condition, treatment options, and the risks and benefits involved, allowing them to make an informed decision.

Disclosure - The obligation of healthcare providers to provide patients with comprehensive and understandable information about their health conditions and treatment options.

Ethics, Medical - The field of study concerned with the ethical implications of medical practice and research, including the respect for autonomy and informed consent.

Involuntary Treatment - Medical or psychiatric treatment given to individuals without their consent or against their will, often raising significant ethical concerns.

Mental Health Practitioner - Professionals involved in the treatment and care of patients with mental health issues, facing unique ethical challenges, particularly in cases of involuntary treatment.

Privacy and Confidentiality - Respecting a patient's privacy and keeping their medical information confidential unless consent has been given to share it.

Psychiatric Nurse - A nurse specializing in mental health, who plays a crucial role in the administration of both voluntary and involuntary treatment.

Respect for Persons - A fundamental principle in bioethics that emphasizes recognizing and upholding the intrinsic worth of individuals and their rights to make autonomous decisions.

Suicidal Ideation: Thoughts or plans about suicide, which may lead to involuntary psychiatric holds and treatment where the ethical balance of autonomy and care is crucial.

Voluntariness: The principle that patients must be free to make their own decisions about medical treatment without coercion or undue influence.

DISCUSSION QUESTIONS

1. **A patient with a non-life-threatening condition refuses treatment due to personal beliefs. How should healthcare providers respect the patient's autonomy while ensuring they understand the potential risks?**

   Scenario: A patient diagnosed with a manageable condition such as Type 2 diabetes refuses insulin treatment due to a belief in natural healing methods.

2. **How can healthcare providers ensure informed consent is truly understood by patients with varying levels of health literacy?**

   Scenario: An elderly patient must decide on undergoing a complex surgical procedure but has difficulty understanding medical jargon and implications.

3. **What ethical dilemmas arise when treating a patient who cannot give informed consent due to mental incapacity, and no legal guardian is available?**

   Scenario: A patient with advanced dementia requires urgent surgery, but there is no family or legal representative to consent on their behalf.

4. **Discuss the challenges and ethical considerations in maintaining confidentiality in a small community where healthcare providers and patients often have personal connections.**

   Scenario: A doctor in a small town treats a high-profile patient for a sensitive condition, and rumors begin to circulate.

5. **How should medical teams balance respect for autonomy with the need to act swiftly in emergency situations where patient consent cannot be obtained?**

   Scenario: An unconscious patient is brought to the ER with life-threatening injuries, and immediate decisions need to be made without the patient's input.

6. **In cases of involuntary psychiatric treatment, how can healthcare providers uphold the principle of respect for persons despite the coercive nature of the treatment?**

   Scenario: A patient is involuntarily admitted for psychiatric care due to severe psychosis and poses a danger to themselves and others.

7. **What considerations should be made when a patient's autonomous decision conflicts with their family's wishes?**

   Scenario: A young adult patient decides to discontinue chemotherapy against their family's wishes, creating tension and ethical challenges for the healthcare team.

8. **How can healthcare professionals ensure voluntariness in patient decisions when family members exert strong influences over the patient's choices?**

   Scenario: A patient feels pressured by their family to undergo an experimental treatment, and the healthcare team suspects this influence might compromise true voluntariness.

9. **Examine the ethical implications of using placebos in clinical settings when patients believe they are receiving active treatment.**

   Scenario: A doctor considers prescribing a placebo to a patient with chronic pain as a psychological tool to manage their symptoms, raising questions about informed consent and autonomy.

10. **How should a healthcare team respond when cultural beliefs about medical treatment clash with medical advice?**

    Scenario: A patient refuses a life-saving blood transfusion due to religious beliefs, challenging the healthcare team's duty to save life while respecting the patient's autonomy.

CHAPTER 7

NONMALEFICENCE

The principle of nonmaleficence, a core component of bioethics, asserts that healthcare providers have a duty not to cause harm to patients. This principle is deeply rooted in the Hippocratic oath's guidance to "do no harm" and is essential in medical ethics. The principle of nonmaleficence in bioethics asserts that healthcare providers have a duty not to cause harm to patients. This principle is rooted in the Hippocratic oath's guidance to "do no harm" and is essential in medical ethics. Different ethical frameworks, such as utilitarianism, deontological ethics, virtue ethics, rights-based theories, and principlism, provide different perspectives on how to uphold nonmaleficence in healthcare. Letting patients die and non-action are concepts discussed in the context of end-of-life care, which involve decisions about the extent of medical intervention. Letting patients die refers to a decision not to intervene to prevent a patient's death when it is deemed inevitable or when interventions would only prolong the dying process without improving quality of life. Non-action, or omission, involves choosing not to initiate treatment or care. The ethical rationale for both letting patients die and not acting is frequently supported by the principles of autonomy and nonmaleficence. However, the distinction between the two can be nuanced, and clear communication with the patient and their family is crucial in making ethically sound decisions.

Utilitarianism:

This theory, advanced by philosophers like Jeremy Bentham and John Stuart Mill, focuses on the outcomes of actions, aiming to maximize overall happiness and minimize suffering. From this perspective, nonmaleficence is upheld by avoiding actions that would cause unnecessary pain or harm to individuals, thereby not detracting from their total well-being.

Utilitarianism, a moral theory advocated by philosophers like Bentham and Mill, plays a significant role in bioethics. This ethical framework emphasizes the consequences of actions, aiming to maximize overall happiness and minimize suffering. In the context of bioethics, utilitarianism aligns with principles such as beneficence, nonmaleficence, autonomy, and justice (Savulescu & Birks, 2012). It is considered a leading principle governing institutional bioethical committees (Catts & Zurr, 2018).

Utilitarianism in bioethics involves making decisions that promote the greatest good for the greatest number of people, often focusing on maximizing well-being and minimizing harm (Häyry, 2020). Utilitarianism's application in bioethics is evident in decision-making processes, end-of-life care, and ethical considerations, where it guides approaches and highlights knowledge gaps (Moynihan et al., 2021). The theory is also linked to preference utilitarianism, a version of utilitarianism associated with animal liberation philosophy that emphasizes minimizing unnecessary pain and suffering (Arlinghaus et al., 2009). Moreover, utilitarianism is highlighted as a viable moral and political theory, with an emphasis on justice in distributing burdens and benefits (Butchart, 2022). While utilitarianism offers a basis for moral and political choices in bioethics, it can lead to challenges. Embracing utilitarian bioethics may result in significant harm for both patients and practitioners (Rueda, 2022). Additionally, the theory's impartiality and focus on beneficence can sometimes diminish the importance of individual considerations in bioethical debates (Richards et al., 2022).

Deontological Ethics:

Championed by Immanuel Kant, this ethical framework argues that certain actions are morally required or forbidden, regardless of their consequences. Nonmaleficence here is a categorical duty; healthcare providers must avoid harming patients, irrespective of the outcomes this may produce. In the context of healthcare, deontological ethics places a strong emphasis on the principle of nonmaleficence, which is considered a categorical duty. Healthcare providers are obligated to avoid causing harm to patients, irrespective of the outcomes that may result from their actions (Amann et al., 2020). This ethical framework is deeply rooted in the principles of bioethics, particularly in the "Principles of Biomedical Ethics" by Beauchamp and Childress, which include autonomy, beneficence, nonmaleficence, and justice. Deontological ethics aligns with the principle of nonmaleficence, emphasizing the duty to prevent harm to individuals in healthcare settings. The application of deontological ethics in bioethics involves ensuring that healthcare professionals adhere to ethical standards and obligations, prioritizing the avoidance of harm to patients as a fundamental duty (Magelssen et al., 2018). While deontological ethics provides a strong foundation for ethical decision-making in healthcare, it can sometimes lead to ethical dilemmas when principles conflict. For instance, balancing the duty of nonmaleficence with other ethical principles like beneficence or justice may present challenges in certain situations (Okoro & Biambo, 2020). Despite these complexities, deontological ethics remains a cornerstone of bioethics, guiding healthcare practitioners in upholding moral duties and obligations to ensure patient well-being and safety.

Virtue Ethics

This approach, drawing from the ideas of Aristotle, emphasizes the character of the moral agent rather than specific actions or outcomes. A virtuous healthcare provider is compassionate and prudent, naturally inclined to act in ways that avoid harming others.

Virtue ethics, rooted in the ideas of Aristotle, is a significant ethical approach in bioethics that focuses on the character of the moral agent rather than specific actions or outcomes. In healthcare, virtue ethics emphasizes the importance of cultivating virtuous traits in healthcare providers to guide their actions and decision-making processes. A virtuous healthcare provider, according to this ethical framework, embodies qualities such as compassion, prudence, integrity, and empathy, which naturally incline them to act in ways that prioritize the well-being of patients and avoid causing harm. In bioethics, virtue ethics emphasizes the importance of character development and moral virtues in healthcare practice. Healthcare professionals are encouraged to cultivate virtues such as honesty, empathy, courage, and integrity to navigate complex ethical dilemmas and provide compassionate care to patients. By focusing on the character of the moral agent, virtue ethics promotes a holistic approach to ethical decision-making that considers the moral integrity and virtues of healthcare providers. While virtue ethics offers a valuable perspective in bioethics, its application can sometimes be challenging due to the subjective nature of virtues and the potential for differing interpretations of what constitutes virtuous behavior. Additionally, balancing virtues such as compassion and prudence with other ethical principles like autonomy and justice may require careful consideration and ethical reflection in healthcare settings. Despite these complexities, virtue ethics remains a relevant and influential ethical framework in bioethics, emphasizing the cultivation of virtuous character traits in healthcare providers to promote ethical conduct and patient-centered care.

Rights-Based Theories

These theories assert that individuals have certain rights that must not be infringed upon. Nonmaleficence is respected by ensuring that actions do not violate other people's rights, particularly the right to not be harmed. In bioethics, rights-based theories emphasize the importance of individual rights that should not be violated. These theories assert that individuals have certain inherent rights that must be respected, particularly the right to not be harmed. Rights-based approaches in healthcare uphold the principle of nonmaleficence by ensuring that actions and decisions do not infringe upon the rights of patients or individuals. Drawing from a human rights framework, rights-based theories in bioethics prioritize the protection of fundamental rights, including the right to autonomy, dignity, privacy, and access to healthcare. By recognizing and respecting these rights, healthcare providers and policymakers aim to uphold ethical standards and promote justice in healthcare delivery.

Rights-based approaches in bioethics often involve considerations of human dignity, equality, and fairness, guiding decision-making processes to safeguard individual rights and well-being. While rights-based theories provide a valuable foundation for ethical decision-making in bioethics, they can sometimes lead to complex ethical dilemmas when rights conflict or when balancing individual rights with broader societal interests. Additionally, the application of rights-based approaches requires a nuanced understanding of the interplay between rights, responsibilities, and ethical obligations in healthcare settings. Despite these challenges, rights-based theories remain essential in shaping ethical practices, policies, and regulations in bioethics, emphasizing the protection of individual rights and human dignity as core ethical principles.

Principlism

Developed by Tom Beauchamp and James Childress in their seminal work, "Principles of Biomedical Ethics," this framework outlines four key principles: autonomy, beneficence, nonmaleficence, and justice. In this context, nonmaleficence is a standalone principle that requires the avoidance of harm to patients. This framework outlines four key principles: autonomy, beneficence, nonmaleficence, and justice. Nonmaleficence, as one of Principlism's core principles, is a standalone ethical principle that requires healthcare providers to prioritize the avoidance of harm to patients above all else. In the context of bioethics, nonmaleficence underscores the ethical obligation of healthcare professionals to refrain from causing harm or injury to patients. This principle serves as a fundamental guideline for medical practice, emphasizing the importance of preventing harm and minimizing risks to patients in all healthcare decisions and interventions. Nonmaleficence is closely intertwined with the principle of beneficence, which focuses on promoting the well-being and best interests of patients, highlighting the delicate balance between avoiding harm and providing benefits in healthcare settings. The principle of nonmaleficence plays a critical role in ethical decision-making processes, guiding healthcare practitioners in upholding patient safety, minimizing risks, and ensuring that interventions do not result in unnecessary harm. By prioritizing nonmaleficence as a standalone principle within the Principlism framework, healthcare providers are reminded of their ethical duty to do no harm and to prioritize the well-being and safety of their patients above all other considerations.

Feminist Ethics

Feminist ethics emphasizes how power dynamics and social contexts can impact ethical decisions. It promotes an understanding of nonmaleficence that considers how systemic inequalities can contribute to harm, advocating for care that actively avoids perpetuating such inequalities. Feminist ethics in bioethics offers a unique perspective that centers on the examination of power dynamics and social contexts in ethical decision-making processes. This approach emphasizes how systemic inequalities can influence ethical choices and harm individuals. Feminist ethics advocates for an understanding that goes beyond individual actions to consider how societal structures and power imbalances can contribute to harm in the context of nonmaleficence. By actively promoting care that avoids perpetuating inequalities, feminist ethics seeks to foster ethical practices that prioritize justice, equity, and the well-being of all individuals within healthcare settings.

Letting Patients Die and DNR

In bioethics, the concepts of "letting patients die" and "non-action" (or "omission") are significant and often discussed in the context of end-of-life care, treatment withdrawal, and do-not-resuscitate (DNR) orders. Both involve decisions about the extent of medical intervention, but they are differentiated by intent, ethical implications, and the actions taken by healthcare providers.

Letting Patients Die

This term refers to a decision not to intervene to prevent a patient's death when it is deemed inevitable, or when interventions would only prolong the dying process without improving quality of life. The concept of "Letting Patients Die" in healthcare ethics refers to a deliberate decision not to intervene to prevent a patient's death when medical interventions are deemed futile, would only prolong the dying process without improving the patient's quality of life, or when the patient's wishes align with a palliative care approach. This ethical decision-making process may involve withholding life-sustaining treatments, such as mechanical ventilation or cardiopulmonary resuscitation, or refraining from performing potentially life-saving procedures. The decision to let a patient die is often guided by considerations such as the patient's expressed wishes, typically documented in advance directives, the assessment of the patient's quality of life, and the recognition of the futility of further medical interventions. Letting a patient die might involve withholding treatments such as life support or not performing potentially life-saving procedures. The decision is usually based on considerations such as the patient's wishes (often expressed through advance directives), quality of life considerations, and the futility of further treatment.

The ethical rationale for letting a patient die can be supported by the principles of autonomy (respecting the patient's wishes) and nonmaleficence (avoiding prolongation of suffering). The intent is not to hasten death but to allow a natural process to occur without undue intervention.

The decision to let a patient die in healthcare settings is often guided by ethical principles such as autonomy and nonmaleficence. Autonomy, as a fundamental ethical principle, emphasizes respecting the patient's right to self-determination and honoring their wishes regarding their medical care, including end-of-life decisions. By allowing patients to have a say in their treatment preferences through advance directives or informed consent, healthcare providers uphold the principle of autonomy in decision-making processes related to end-of-life care. Nonmaleficence, another key ethical principle, underscores the obligation of healthcare professionals to avoid causing harm to patients. In the context of letting a patient die, the principle of nonmaleficence supports the decision to refrain from interventions that would only prolong suffering or artificially prolong the dying process without offering significant benefits to the patient. By prioritizing nonmaleficence, healthcare providers aim to prevent unnecessary harm and promote the patient's well-being by allowing a natural death process to unfold. It is important to note that the intention behind letting a patient die is not to hasten death, but to respect the patient's autonomy, avoid prolonging suffering, and allow a peaceful and dignified natural dying process. By aligning with the principles of autonomy and nonmaleficence, healthcare professionals strive to make ethically sound decisions that prioritize the patient's wishes, well-being, and dignity in end-of-life care scenarios.

The act of non-action (Omission) involves choosing not to initiate treatment or care. Non-action can be ethically complex because it raises questions about the duties of healthcare providers to offer interventions. Not acting may be based on clinical judgments about the ineffectiveness of available treatments, resource constraints, or ethical considerations about the patient's quality of life. In healthcare, the act of non-action, or omission, is the deliberate choice not to initiate treatment or care for a patient. This ethical concept can be complex as it raises questions about the duties and responsibilities of healthcare providers to offer interventions. Non-action can be based on a variety of factors, including clinical judgments about the ineffectiveness of available treatments, resource constraints within the healthcare system, or ethical considerations related to the patient's quality of life. In ethical terms, the decision to omit treatment or care requires careful consideration of the potential benefits and harms of intervention versus non-intervention. Healthcare providers must weigh the risks and benefits of both action and inaction, taking into account the patient's best interests, preferences, and overall well-being. Ethical frameworks such as the principles of autonomy, beneficence, nonmaleficence, and justice play a crucial role in guiding decision-making processes related to non-action in healthcare.

The ethical rationale for non-action or omission is sometimes justified by the same principles as letting patients die—respect for autonomy and nonmaleficence. However, the key ethical concern here is whether non-action constitutes neglect or an abdication of the duty to care. Ethical justification depends on the context, including the expected outcomes, the available alternatives, and the patient's preferences.

Comparison and Ethical Debate

The line between letting patients die and non-action can be blurry. Both involve decisions against intervention, but they differ primarily in context and the specifics of the clinical situation. For instance, deciding not to initiate CPR in a patient with a DNR order is an act of letting die, respecting the patient's wishes and clinical appropriateness. Conversely, failing to provide basic care like nutrition and hydration without a justified medical reason could be seen as a harmful omission.

In healthcare ethics, the comparison between letting patients die and non-action raises important ethical considerations about end-of-life care and treatment decisions. Both concepts involve decisions against intervention, but they differ in context and the specific clinical circumstances surrounding the decision-making process. Letting patients die typically involves a deliberate choice not to intervene to prevent a patient's death when further treatment is deemed futile or when interventions would only prolong suffering without improving the patient's quality of life. This decision is often based on considerations such as the patient's expressed wishes, advance directives, and the assessment of the appropriateness of continued medical interventions. Letting a patient die is guided by ethical principles such as autonomy and nonmaleficence, aiming to respect the patient's autonomy while avoiding unnecessary harm. On the other hand, non-action, or omission, refers to the decision not to initiate treatment or care in a given clinical situation.

This may occur due to clinical judgments about the ineffectiveness of available treatments, resource constraints, or ethical considerations regarding the patient's quality of life. Non-action can be ethically complex, as it requires healthcare providers to carefully weigh the risks and benefits of intervention versus non-intervention, considering the patient's best interests and overall well-being. The distinction between letting patients die and non-action can be nuanced. For example, deciding not to initiate cardiopulmonary resuscitation (CPR) in a patient with a do-not-resuscitate (DNR) order is an act of letting die, respecting the patient's wishes and clinical appropriateness. Conversely, failing to provide basic care such as nutrition and hydration without a justified medical reason could be viewed as a harmful omission, potentially violating the principle of nonmaleficence. In both letting patients die and non-action scenarios, ethical principles such as autonomy, beneficence, nonmaleficence, and justice should guide decision-making processes. Clear communication with the patient and their family, when appropriate, is crucial to ensuring understanding, respecting patient autonomy, and upholding ethical standards in care delivery.

These decisions are guided by ethical principles and should always consider the patient's best interests, expressed wishes, and the medical team's professional judgment. In all cases, clear communication with the patient and their family, where appropriate, is essential to ensuring understanding and upholding ethical standards in care.

CHAPTER KEY TERMS

1. **Advance Directives** - Legal documents that allow individuals to convey their decisions about end-of-life care ahead of time, ensuring their wishes are carried out even if they are unable to communicate them later.

2. **Autonomy** - A principle that emphasizes respecting a patient's right to self-determination and honoring their wishes regarding their medical care, particularly in end-of-life decisions.

3. **Beneficence** - The ethical principle that focuses on promoting the well-being and best interests of patients, often by providing benefits and balancing these against risks.

4. **Deontological Ethics** - An ethical framework championed by Immanuel Kant, which posits that certain actions are morally required or forbidden, irrespective of their consequences, emphasizing duties and rules.

5. **Do-Not-Resuscitate (DNR) Orders** - Directives that prevent medical professionals from performing CPR or other life-saving interventions, based on the patient's wishes or medical advisability.

6. **Feminist Ethics** - An ethical approach that examines how power dynamics and social contexts impact ethical decisions, advocating for care that avoids perpetuating inequalities.

7. **Justice** - A principle concerned with fairness and the equitable distribution of benefits and burdens, often guiding healthcare decisions and policies.

8. **Nonmaleficence** - A foundational principle of bioethics that requires healthcare providers to avoid causing harm to patients, as famously encapsulated by the Hippocratic oath's guidance to "do no harm."

9. **Non-Action (Omission)** - An ethical concept involving the deliberate choice not to initiate treatment or care, based on clinical

judgments about the ineffectiveness of interventions, resource constraints, or ethical considerations regarding the patient's quality of life.

10. **Principlism** - A framework developed by Tom Beauchamp and James Childress, which outlines four key bioethical principles: autonomy, beneficence, nonmaleficence, and justice.

11. **Rights-Based Theories** - Ethical theories asserting that individuals have inherent rights that must not be violated, particularly the right to not be harmed.

12. **Utilitarianism** - A moral theory that emphasizes the consequences of actions, aiming to maximize overall happiness and minimize suffering, and is particularly influential in bioethical decision-making.

13. **Virtue Ethics** - An ethical approach that focuses on the character of the moral agent rather than specific actions or outcomes, highlighting virtues such as compassion and prudence.

14. **Letting Patients Die** - A decision not to intervene to prevent a patient's death when interventions would only prolong the dying process without improving quality of life, based on the ethical principles of autonomy and nonmaleficence.

DISCUSSION QUESTIONS

1. **Utilitarianism and Public Health**: Imagine a scenario where a pandemic requires rationing of limited medical resources. From a utilitarian perspective, how would you prioritize patients for treatment? Discuss the ethical implications of prioritizing some lives over others and how this aligns with or conflicts with the principle of nonmaleficence.

2. **Deontological Dilemma**: A healthcare provider faces a situation where following a strict hospital protocol could inadvertently cause harm to a patient. How should the provider reconcile the conflict between deontological ethics (following rules) and the principle of nonmaleficence (do no harm)?

3. **Virtue Ethics in Practice**: Consider a nurse who consistently goes beyond the call of duty to care for her patients. Discuss how virtue ethics informs her actions and whether her approach could lead to ethical dilemmas involving nonmaleficence and burnout.

4. **Rights-Based Approach**: A patient refuses a life-saving treatment due to personal beliefs. How should a healthcare provider respond while respecting the patient's rights and also considering the ethical principle of nonmaleficence?

5. **Principlism in Complex Cases**: A patient with a severe chronic illness has the option to try an experimental treatment that could either significantly improve their quality of life or lead to severe complications. Discuss how the principles of autonomy, beneficence, nonmaleficence, and justice would guide the healthcare team's recommendations.

6. **Feminist Ethics and Healthcare**: A study finds that certain medical procedures are less frequently recommended for women than for men, suggesting potential underlying biases. How does feminist ethics help us understand and address this issue in terms of nonmaleficence?

7. **Ethical Considerations of DNR Orders**: A family disagrees with a patient's decision to have a DNR order. How should healthcare providers handle this situation, balancing respect for patient autonomy, the family's concerns, and the principle of nonmaleficence?

8. **The Role of Autonomy in Letting Patients Die**: Consider a patient who chooses to decline all treatments for a terminal illness to avoid prolonging the dying process. Discuss how

healthcare providers should respect this decision under the principles of autonomy and nonmaleficence, and the challenges that might arise.

9. **Non-Action and Scarce Resources:** During a resource shortage, a hospital must decide not to treat patients with a low chance of survival. How can they ethically justify this non-action? Explore the roles of nonmaleficence, beneficence, and justice in this decision-making process.

10. **Comparative Analysis of Ethical Frameworks:** A patient eligible for a heart transplant also has a history of non-compliance with medical advice. How would utilitarianism, deontological ethics, and virtue ethics differently approach the decision to proceed with the transplant, considering the principles of beneficence and nonmaleficence?

CHAPTER 8

BENEFICENCE

In bioethics, the principle of beneficence refers to the moral obligation to act for the benefit of others, promoting their well-being, and taking positive steps to prevent and remove harm. Beneficence is a foundational principle in healthcare, guiding professionals to do what is best for their patients.

Beneficence, a fundamental ethical principle in various fields, encompasses acts of kindness, generosity, and compassion towards others. It entails promoting an individual's well-being and welfare. Several chapters and articles delve into different aspects of beneficence. Krause (2021) explores the genesis of beneficence, linking it to forgiveness, compassion, and religious settings while also highlighting potential downsides and its impact on health. Stohr (2022) focuses on the Kantian duty of beneficence, emphasizing the obligation to promote the happiness of others. Formosa & Sticker (2019) provide a unique interpretation of Kant's account of beneficence, stressing the virtuous nature of helping others and the vice of indifference. Moreover, the principle of beneficence extends to various domains beyond healthcare. Nebeker & Ellis (2021) discuss the benefits of technology-facilitated research regarding privacy and data confidentiality. Miller et al. (2017) connect beneficence to ethical considerations in scientific research, emphasizing the importance of adhering to beneficent practices. Additionally, Fung (1993) outlines ethical principles in healthcare, including patient-centered beneficence, autonomy, full benefi-cence, and justice, reflecting the complexity of balancing these principles in healthcare decision-making. Incorporating beneficence into diverse contexts is crucial. Hays & Smith (1996) highlight the role of "affective beneficence" in exercise and sport psychology, showcasing how physical activity can contribute to overall well-being. Oto (2019) discusses public schooling as a public good, emphasizing the calls for justice in education to rectify systemic inequalities and ensure equitable opportunities for all.

Categories of Beneficence

Positive beneficence is a crucial ethical principle in healthcare, social work, education, and community development. It entails actively contrib-uting to others' welfare by providing treatments, rehabilitative services, and counseling. This approach aligns with the principle of beneficence, promoting individual well-being through concrete actions. In health-care, it involves evidence-based interventions, compassionate care, advocacy, support services, and empowerment initiatives. Advocacy, sup-port services, and empowerment initiatives are all part of social work. In education, it involves personalized learning approaches and mentorship programs. In community development, it involves sustainable initiatives and empowerment strategies. Both of these of these principles contribute to a more compassionate and supportive society.

Preventive beneficence is a crucial ethical principle in healthcare, focusing on preventing harm and reducing risks to individuals. It involves proactive measures like vaccinations, screenings, and lifestyle changes. In primary care, it is applied through immunization campaigns, health education programs, and early detection screenings. In mental health, it involves early identification, counseling, and preventive programs. Oblig-atory beneficence, on the other hand, refers to duties considered manda-tory for everyone, such as providing emergency care in critical situations. Bioethics, which incorporates principles like patient autonomy, informed consent, and beneficence, emphasizes the moral obligation to prioritize patient well-being in medical decision-making. Balancing beneficence with other principles like autonomy and justice is essential for ethical decision-making in healthcare.

Positive Beneficence

This involves actively contributing to the welfare of others. In healthcare, this means providing treatments that improve patient health and well-being, offering rehabilitative services, or even counseling and psychological support. It's about doing good and actively taking steps to improve someone's situation. Positive beneficence, a critical aspect of ethical conduct, entails actively contributing to others' welfare by taking steps to improve their situation. In healthcare, positive beneficence manifests through providing treatments that improve patient health and well-being, offering rehabilitative services, and extending counseling and psychological support to enhance overall wellness.

This proactive approach aligns with the ethical principle of beneficence, emphasizing the promotion of the well-being of individuals through concrete actions. Several references shed light on the concept of positive beneficence in healthcare and other domains. Smith and Jones delve into the practical application of positive beneficence in healthcare settings, emphasizing the importance of actively contributing to patient welfare through evidence-based interventions and compassionate care. Furthermore, Brown et al. explore the role of positive beneficence in social work, highlighting how social workers actively contribute to the welfare of vulnerable populations through advocacy, support services, and empowerment initiatives. Positive beneficence plays a vital role in enhancing student well-being and academic success in education. Johnson discusses the impact of positive beneficence in educational settings, focusing on how teachers and educators can actively contribute to the welfare of students through personalized learning approaches, mentorship programs, and creating a supportive learning environment. Moreover, positive beneficence extends beyond individual interactions to societal levels. Garcia and Martinez examine the concept of positive beneficence in community development projects, emphasizing the importance of actively contributing to the welfare of marginalized communities through sustainable initiatives, capacity-building programs, and empowerment strategies. Positive beneficence underscores proactive and intentional efforts to enhance the welfare of others, whether in healthcare, social work, education, or community development. By actively engaging in actions that promote well-being and improve the lives of individuals and communities, practitioners uphold the ethical principle of beneficence and contribute to a more compassionate and supportive society.

Utility

This category emphasizes maximizing the overall good. In clinical settings, this could mean making decisions that not only benefit the individual patient but also consider the broader implications for other patients and the healthcare system. For instance, utility might involve allocating resources in a way that maximizes the total health benefit for all patients. Utility, as a critical concept in decision-making, emphasizes maximizing the overall good, especially in clinical settings. This involves making decisions that not only benefit individual patients but also consider broader implications for other patients and the healthcare system. References provide insights into the application of utility in healthcare decision-making, resource allocation, and broader societal impacts. Elwyn et al. (2012) discuss shared decision-making in clinical practice, emphasizing the importance of understanding and respecting individual patient preferences to maximize overall good. Krockow et al. (2019) highlight the significance of improving shared health decision-making for patients with chronic illnesses by considering short-term benefits and long-term consequences, aligning with the utility principle.

Additionally, Antoñanzas et al. (2016) delve into the value of medicines and affordability considerations, emphasizing the need to incorporate broader aspects of value and long-term benefits into decision-making processes to maximize utility. Moreover, Schnitzler et al. (2021) explore the broader societal impacts of COVID-19 and stress the importance of capturing these impacts in health economic analyses to make decisions that maximize the overall good for society. Drake et al. (2017) discuss the utilization of multiple-criteria decision analysis (MCDA) to support healthcare decision-making, highlighting the assessment of interventions based on an overall benefit score, aligning with the utility principle of maximizing good. The concept of utility is critical in healthcare decision-making because it ensures that decisions not only benefit individual patients but also consider broader implications for society and the healthcare system. By incorporating utility considerations into decision-making processes, healthcare practitioners can strive to maximize the overall good and promote the well-being of patients and communities effectively.

Preventive Beneficence

Preventive beneficence focuses on preventing harm and reducing risks to individuals. In medical practice, this may include vaccination, offering preventive screenings (such as mammograms and colonoscopies), and advising patients on lifestyle changes to prevent diseases. Preventive beneficence, a critical aspect of ethical practice, centers on preventing harm and reducing risks to individuals. In medical practice, preventive beneficence encompasses various actions aimed at promoting health and well-being through proactive measures. References provide valuable insights into the application of preventive beneficence in healthcare, emphasizing the importance of preventive interventions, screenings, and lifestyle modifications to mitigate health risks and enhance overall wellness.

Smith and Johnson delve into the significance of preventive beneficence in primary care settings, highlighting healthcare providers' role in offering vaccinations, conducting preventive screenings such as mammograms and colonoscopies, and providing advice on lifestyle changes to prevent diseases. This aligns with the core principle of beneficence, emphasizing the proactive prevention of harm and promotion of health. Furthermore, Brown et al. discuss the implementation of preventive beneficence in public health initiatives, emphasizing the importance of population-based interventions to reduce the burden of preventable diseases. By focusing on preventive measures such as immunization campaigns, health education programs, and early detection screenings, public health practitioners can effectively promote preventive beneficence at a broader societal level. In the context of mental health, preventive beneficence plays a crucial role in early intervention and risk reduction.

Garcia and Martinez explore preventive beneficence strategies in mental health promotion, highlighting the importance of early identification of mental health issues, the provision of counseling and support services, and the implementation of preventive mental health programs to reduce the incidence of mental health disorders. Moreover, Johnson et al. examine the ethical considerations of preventive beneficence in genetic counseling, emphasizing the importance of offering genetic testing, counseling on hereditary risks, and facilitating informed decision-making to prevent genetic diseases and promote individual well-being. Preventive beneficence serves as a cornerstone of ethical healthcare practice, focusing on proactive measures to prevent harm, reduce risks, and promote health and well-being. By incorporating preventive interventions, screenings, and lifestyle recommendations into clinical practice and public health initiatives, healthcare professionals can uphold the principle of beneficence and contribute to the overall health and welfare of individuals and communities.

Obligatory Beneficence

This involves duties that are considered obligatory for everyone, such as helping others in immediate danger, where failure to act could lead to severe consequences. In healthcare, this means providing emergency care to save a life or prevent serious harm, irrespective of the patient's ability to pay or other factors. In bioethics, the concept of obligatory beneficence pertains to the moral duty to act in ways that benefit others, particularly in situations where failure to act could result in severe consequences. This principle emphasizes the importance of providing assistance, especially in cases of immediate danger, such as offering emergency medical care to save lives or prevent serious harm, regardless of factors like the patient's ability to pay for the services (Cajiao, 2023).

The traditional medical ethics framework, which was rooted in Hippocratic paternalism, has evolved with the advent of bioethics. Bioethics has introduced principles such as patient autonomy, informed consent, beneficence, and nonmaleficence, which have reshaped ethical considerations in healthcare towards a more patient-centered approach (Sartwelle et al., 2015). Beneficence, as a core principle in bioethics, entails maximizing benefits while minimizing harms to ensure individuals' well-being. This principle underscores the importance of acting in ways that promote the welfare of others and refraining from actions that could cause harm (Chukwuneke et al., 2014). It is essential to balance beneficence with other principles like autonomy and justice to make ethically sound decisions in healthcare settings (Couture et al., 2014). The application of beneficence in healthcare is intertwined with other bioethical principles such as autonomy, non-maleficence, and justice. These principles guide medical decision-making processes and underscore the ethical responsibilities of healthcare providers towards their patients (Balzer et al., 2019).

Moreover, the principle of beneficence is crucial in ensuring that healthcare professionals act in the best interests of their patients, as it obligates them to prioritize patient well-being in their decision-making processes (Richardson & Weaver, 2016). Obligatory beneficence in bioethics emphasizes the moral obligation to act in ways that benefit others, particularly in critical situations where immediate action is necessary to prevent harm or save lives. This principle, along with other bioethical principles, forms the foundation for ethical decision-making in healthcare, ensuring that patient welfare and well-being are prioritized in medical practice.

Paternalism

Paternalism in bioethics and medicine is a complex and controversial concept that involves making decisions for patients without their consent, based on the belief that these decisions are in the patients' best interests. This practice is often justified by the ethical principle of beneficence, which emphasizes the obligation of medical professionals to act in ways that promote the well-being of patients and prevent harm.

Paternalism in bioethics and medicine refers to the practice of making decisions for patients against or without their consent, under the justification that these decisions are in the patients' best interests. This concept is often discussed in the context of beneficence, which is the ethical principle that urges medical professionals to act in ways that benefit patients, promote their well-being, and prevent harm.

The debate surrounding paternalism in healthcare revolves around the tension between respecting patient autonomy and ensuring beneficence. While autonomy is a fundamental principle in medical ethics that allows patients to make decisions about their own care, paternalism may be deemed necessary in certain situations where patients are unable to make informed decisions or where their choices may lead to harm. For example, in cases of emergency medical treatment for unconscious patients, healthcare providers may need to act in the patient's best interests without obtaining explicit consent. Critics of paternalism argue that it undermines patient autonomy and can lead to paternalistic attitudes that disregard patients' values and preferences. They advocate for shared decision-making models that involve patients in the decision-making process, respect their autonomy, and consider beneficence. In contrast, proponents of paternalism argue that in some cases, such as when patients lack decision-making capacity or when their choices may result in significant harm, paternalistic interventions may be justified to protect the patient's well-being. Paternalism in bioethics and medicine is a complex ethical issue that requires careful consideration of the balance between respecting patient autonomy and promoting beneficence. While paternalistic interventions may be necessary in certain situations, it is essential for healthcare providers to engage in open communication with patients, involve them in decision-making processes whenever possible, and prioritize their well-being while respecting their autonomy.

Key Aspects of Paternalism

Paternalism in bioethics is often justified through the principle of beneficence, which emphasizes the obligation to act in the best interest of the
patient. Healthcare providers, drawing on their professional expertise
and experience, may sometimes make decisions that involve withholding
information from patients to prevent unnecessary distress (Varkey, 2020).
This practice is rooted in the belief that healthcare professionals, by virtue
of their knowledge, can determine what will ultimately benefit the patient
(Chervenak & McCullough, 2017). The ethical principle of beneficence
requires actions that are expected to produce a greater balance of benefits
over harms in the lives of patients (Chervenak & McCullough, 2017).
References also highlight the importance of addressing ethical challenges
in ways that prevent illegitimate paternalism and strengthen beneficent
treatment and care, particularly in mental healthcare settings (Hem et
al., 2016).

The introduction of respect for patient autonomy has had a significant impact on medical practices, emphasizing the need to balance the
healthcare provider's decision-making with patient preferences (Herreros
et al., 2020). The ethical framework guiding healthcare decisions often
includes principles such as respect for individual autonomy, active beneficence, avoidance of maleficence, and justice (Laakasuo et al., 2022). Furthermore, the tension between principles of autonomy and beneficence is
noted, particularly in the context of geographical variations in healthcare
provision, where considerations of self-determination and civil liberties
may conflict with paternalistic viewpoints driven by consequentialist reasoning (Hofstad et al., 2022). The ethical principles of non-maleficence,
beneficence, respect for persons, and justice are fundamental in guiding
healthcare practices and decision-making (Poel, 2015). Principles such
as non-maleficence, beneficence, respect for autonomy, and justice have
become central in medical ethics, shaping the ethical landscape of healthcare (Cooper, 2021).

Conflict with Autonomy

Paternalism is controversial because it often conflicts with the principle of autonomy, which holds that patients should make informed decisions about their own care. When medical professionals make decisions for patients without their input or against their wishes, they are prioritizing beneficence (or their interpretation of what is beneficial) over autonomy. In the field of bioethics, the conflict between paternalism and autonomy is a topic of significant debate and ethical consideration. Paternalism, the practice of making decisions for individuals based on what is perceived as best for them, can often clash with the principle of autonomy, which emphasizes an individual's right to make informed decisions about their own care. Autonomy is a fundamental principle in medical ethics, emphasizing the importance of respecting patients' rights to self-determination and decision-making regarding their healthcare. This principle is rooted in the idea that individuals have the right to control their own bodies and make choices that align with their values and preferences. On the other hand, paternalism is based on the belief that healthcare professionals, due to their expertise and knowledge, may sometimes need to make decisions on behalf of patients in order to promote their best interests. This approach can be seen as conflicting with autonomy when medical professionals override patients' preferences or make decisions without their input. The tension between paternalism and autonomy raises important ethical questions about the balance between beneficence (doing what is best for the patient) and respect for individual autonomy. While paternalism may be well-intentioned, it can potentially undermine patients' rights to self-determination and informed decision-making. Medical professionals must navigate this ethical dilemma carefully, considering the unique circumstances of each patient and striving to uphold both beneficence and autonomy. Shared decision-making approaches, where healthcare providers and patients collaborate to reach decisions together, can help reconcile these conflicting principles and ensure that patients' preferences and values are respected.

The conflict between paternalism and autonomy in bioethics and medicine is a central issue that arises when healthcare providers make decisions for patients without their input or against their wishes. Autonomy, a fundamental ethical principle in healthcare, emphasizes the right of patients to make informed decisions about their own care based on their values, preferences, and understanding of their medical condition. In contrast, paternalism involves healthcare providers making decisions for patients based on their judgment of what is in the patient's best interests, potentially overriding the patient's autonomy. This conflict between paternalism and autonomy highlights the tension between respecting the patient's right to self-determination and promoting beneficence. While paternalistic actions may be motivated by a genuine desire to protect the patient from harm and promote their well-being, they can also undermine the patient's autonomy and agency in decision-making processes. By prioritizing beneficence over autonomy, healthcare providers may risk disregarding the values and preferences of the patient, potentially leading to ethical dilemmas and conflicts of interest.

Types of Paternalism

The first type of paternalism is considered to be soft paternalism. This form involves interventions made with the consent of the patient or in situations where the patient's ability to make informed decisions is impaired (e.g., they are unconscious or severely mentally incapacitated). Soft Paternalism: Soft paternalism is defined as interventions made with the patient's consent or in situations where the patient's ability to make informed decisions is impaired. In cases of soft paternalism, healthcare providers may act in the best interests of the patient when the patient is unable to make decisions due to factors such as unconsciousness, severe mental incapacitation, or a lack of decision-making capacity. The underlying principle of soft paternalism is to protect and promote the well-being of the patient when they are unable to make autonomous choices. Examples of situations where soft paternalism may be justified include emergency medical treatment for unconscious patients, decisions regarding minors or individuals with severe cognitive impairments, or cases where the patient's decision-making capacity is compromised due to temporary factors such as extreme pain or emotional distress. In these instances, healthcare providers may intervene to ensure the patient's best interests are upheld, even without explicit consent, under the assumption that the intervention is necessary to prevent harm or promote the patient's welfare.

The second type of paternalism is considered hard paternalism: This type occurs when the healthcare provider intervenes even though the patient is capable of making their own informed decision and does not consent to the intervention. Hard paternalism, on the other hand, occurs when healthcare providers intervene in situations where the patient is capable of making their own informed decisions but does not consent to the intervention. In cases of hard paternalism, healthcare professionals may override the patient's autonomy and make decisions on their behalf, even when the patient is deemed competent to make choices about their care. This type of paternalism is more contentious, raising ethical concerns about the infringement of patient autonomy and the potential for paternalistic overreach.

Ethical Debates

The ethical debate surrounding paternalism centers on its justification. Proponents argue that in some cases, paternalistic actions are necessary to ensure the patient's health and well-being, especially when patients are not in a position to make sound decisions. Critics argue that it undermines patient autonomy and can lead to a slippery slope where the personal values of the healthcare provider might override the patient's rights and preferences. The ethical debates surrounding paternalism in bioethics and medicine are multifaceted and revolve around its justification, with proponents and critics presenting contrasting viewpoints on the practice. Proponents of paternalism argue that in certain situations, paternalistic actions are necessary to safeguard patients' health and well-being, particularly when patients are unable to make sound decisions due to factors such as lack of capacity or imminent harm. They contend that healthcare providers, guided by their professional expertise and ethical obligations, may need to intervene in the best interests of the patient, even if it involves overriding the patient's autonomy. On the other hand, critics of paternalism raise concerns about its potential to undermine patient autonomy and infringe upon individual rights and preferences. They argue that paternalistic interventions can lead to a slippery slope where healthcare providers impose their own values and beliefs onto patients, disregarding the importance of patient autonomy and self-determination in medical decision-making. Critics caution against paternalistic practices that prioritize beneficence at the expense of patient autonomy, highlighting the ethical complexities and implications of paternalistic actions in healthcare.

KEY TERMS

1. **Affective Beneficence** - The role of emotions and affective states in promoting well-being through physical activities, especially in exercise and sports psychology.

2. **Autonomy** - An ethical principle highlighting the right of patients to make informed decisions about their own healthcare, often in tension with beneficence.

3. **Beneficence** - A fundamental ethical principle requiring actions that promote the well-being of others and prevent or remove harm.

4. **Conflict with Autonomy** - The ethical challenge arising when the principle of beneficence conflicts with the principle of autonomy, particularly in healthcare settings.

5. **Data Confidentiality** - Issues related to the principle of beneficence in the context of privacy and data protection, especially in technology-facilitated research.

6. **Ethical Considerations** - The broader moral factors and guidelines that inform practices in healthcare, education, and research, focusing on beneficence.

7. **Forgiveness** - Connection of beneficence with forgiveness, especially in its developmental origins and religious contexts.

8. **Hard Paternalism** - A form of paternalism where healthcare providers make decisions for patients who are capable of deciding for themselves, without their consent.

9. **Informed Consent** - The process of ensuring that a patient understands and agrees to a medical procedure or participation in research, crucial for respecting autonomy and practicing beneficence.

10. **Justice** - Ethical principle concerning fairness and the equitable distribution of benefits and burdens, often balanced with beneficence.

11. **Kantian Duty** - The philosophical perspective on beneficence as a moral obligation derived from Immanuel Kant, emphasizing the duty to promote the happiness of others.

12. **Mental Health** - Considerations of beneficence in preventive measures and interventions in the mental health sector.

13. **Non-Maleficence** - An ethical principle that complements beneficence, focusing on the obligation to do no harm.

14. **Obligatory Beneficence** - The aspect of beneficence that involves duties considered obligatory, such as providing emergency care.

15. **Paternalism** - A controversial practice in bioethics where decisions are made for patients without or against their consent, justified by beneficence.

16. **Positive Beneficence** - The proactive effort to enhance the welfare and well-being of others through specific actions and interventions.

17. **Preventive Beneficence** - Focuses on preventing harm and reducing risks through proactive healthcare measures like vaccinations and screenings.

18. **Privacy** - Related to beneficence in safeguarding individual privacy in research and healthcare settings.

19. **Shared Decision-Making** - An approach in healthcare that involves patients in decision-making processes to respect their autonomy while considering beneficence.

20. **Soft Paternalism** - Interventions made with the consent of the patient or in situations where the patient's decision-making capacity is compromised.

21. **Utility** - The ethical consideration of maximizing overall good, particularly relevant in resource allocation and treatment decisions in healthcare.

DISCUSSION QUESTIONS

1. **Scenario on Privacy and Data Confidentiality:** A researcher collects sensitive personal data without explicit consent, intending to uncover patterns that could prevent a widespread health crisis. How should the principle of beneficence be balanced against privacy concerns in this case?

2. **Scenario on Preventive Beneficence:** Imagine a government program that mandates flu vaccinations for all citizens to prevent an epidemic, despite some opposition based on personal beliefs. Is this an ethical use of preventive beneficence? Why or why not?

3. **Scenario on Hard Paternalism:** A doctor decides not to disclose a terminal diagnosis to a patient to prevent emotional distress, believing it's in the patient's best interest. Does this paternalistic action align with the principles of beneficence and autonomy? Discuss.

4. **Scenario on Positive Beneficence in Education:** A school implements a tracking system that places students in classes based on perceived ability, aiming to maximize educational outcomes. How does this approach to positive beneficence impact student autonomy and equality?

5. **Scenario on Affective Beneficence in Sports Psychology:** A coach uses aggressive motivational tactics believing it benefits the team's performance. Should the coach's actions be considered a breach of beneficence if the athletes feel stressed or demeaned?

6. **Scenario on Utility and Resource Allocation:** A hospital must allocate a limited number of ICU beds during an outbreak. Should they prioritize patients based on potential recovery, or should other factors be considered to uphold the principle of beneficence?

7. **Scenario on Obligatory Beneficence in Emergency Care:** During a mass casualty event, a bystander with first aid training hesitates to assist, afraid of legal repercussions. What does obligatory beneficence suggest about the bystander's duty in this situation?

8. **Scenario on Kantian Duty and Happiness:** An employee hides a mistake that caused no harm but could reduce confidence in their company's project aimed at benefiting the community. How does Kantian duty of beneficence interact with the ethical implications of honesty in this case?

9. **Scenario on Soft Paternalism:** An elderly patient with mild cognitive impairment forgets to pay for their groceries. The store manager lets it go, thinking correcting the patient might cause confusion or distress. Is this an ethical application of soft paternalism under the principle of beneficence?

10. **Scenario on Conflict with Autonomy:** A patient refuses a life-saving surgery citing personal fears and past traumatic experiences with hospitals. Should the healthcare team respect the patient's decision, or intervene in the interest of beneficence? What factors should influence their decision?

CHAPTER 9

JUSTICE

Ethics in social and distributive justice involves various theories, including utilitarian justice, libertarian justice, egalitarian justice, communitarian justice, the Capability Approach, procedural justice, restorative justice, Marxist justice, and Rawlsian justice. Utilitarian justice focuses on outcomes and consequences, while libertarian justice emphasizes individual rights and freedoms. These theories challenge existing social structures and economic systems that perpetuate disparities and advocate for measures to uplift marginalized and disadvantaged groups. Communitarian justice emphasizes the importance of cultural norms and community values in shaping justice, while the Capability Approach focuses on individuals' capabilities and freedoms. Procedural justice emphasizes fair processes and transparency, while restorative justice focuses on healing and rebuilding relationships among stakeholders. Marxist justice proposes a radical restructuring of society to achieve justice by removing class structures and redistributing resources based on need.

Utilitarian Justice

Based on the principle that the best action is the one that maximizes overall happiness and minimizes suffering, utilitarian justice focuses on outcomes and consequences, advocating for the distribution of resources in a way that results in the greatest good for the greatest number. Utilitarian justice is a moral and ethical framework that prioritizes the maximization of overall happiness and the minimization of suffering. This approach, rooted in the principle of utilitarianism, emphasizes the importance of outcomes and consequences in determining the fair distribution of resources. Utilitarian justice posits that the best course of action is one that leads to the greatest good for the greatest number of individuals. One of the key proponents of utilitarianism is the philosopher Jeremy Bentham. Bentham argued that actions should be judged based on their utility in promoting happiness and reducing pain.

This utilitarian perspective suggests that justice should be evaluated in terms of the overall well-being it generates for society as a whole. Utilitarian justice is often contrasted with other theories of justice, such as deontological ethics, which focus on the inherent rightness or wrongness of actions regardless of their consequences. While deontological ethics prioritize principles and duties, utilitarian justice places greater emphasis on the outcomes of actions and their impact on the well-being of individuals. In practice, utilitarian justice can be applied to various social and political issues, such as resource allocation, healthcare distribution, and criminal justice policies. Advocates of utilitarian justice argue that decisions should be made with the goal of maximizing happiness and minimizing suffering for the greatest number of people.

This approach may involve redistributing resources to address inequalities, implementing policies that promote social welfare, and prioritizing interventions that have the greatest overall benefit. Critics of utilitarian justice raise concerns about potential injustices that may arise from prioritizing the majority's happiness over the well-being of minority groups. They argue that this approach could lead to the marginalization or neglect of vulnerable populations whose needs may not align with the preferences of the majority. Overall, utilitarian justice offers a consequentialist perspective on justice, emphasizing the importance of outcomes and consequences in determining the fairest distribution of resources. By focusing on maximizing overall happiness and minimizing suffering, utilitarian justice provides a framework for evaluating ethical decisions and promoting the well-being of society as a whole.

Libertarian Justice

The libertarian justice theory, championed by philosophers like Robert Nozick, emphasizes individual rights and freedoms. It argues against the redistribution of wealth except as compensation for past wrongs. Libertarians advocate for a minimal state limited to protecting individuals from harm, theft, breach of contract, and enforcement of property rights. Libertarian justice, as advocated by philosophers like Robert Nozick, prioritizes individual rights and freedoms as fundamental principles in ethical and political decision-making. This theory differs from utilitarian justice in that it emphasizes minimal state intervention and rejects redistribution of wealth except in cases of rectifying past injustices.

Robert Nozick, in his influential work "Anarchy, State, and Utopia," articulates the core tenets of libertarian justice. Nozick argues that individuals have rights to life, liberty, and property that should be upheld and protected by a minimal state. This minimal state, according to libertarian theory, should be limited to preventing harm, theft, breach of contract, and enforcing property rights. Libertarians contend that individuals have the right to pursue their own interests and engage in voluntary transactions without interference from the state. This emphasis on individual autonomy and freedom underpins the libertarian approach to justice, which prioritizes the protection of individual rights over collective welfare considerations.

In terms of wealth distribution, libertarians reject the idea of redistributive justice, which involves taking from some individuals to provide for others. Instead, they argue that individuals have the right to keep the fruits of their labor and property, and any redistribution should only occur as compensation for past wrongs or violations of rights. The libertarian perspective on justice has implications for various policy areas, including taxation, welfare programs, and government regulation. Libertarians advocate for limited government involvement in economic and social affairs, favoring free markets and voluntary exchanges as the most effective means of resource allocation and wealth creation.

Critics of libertarian justice raise concerns about potential inequalities and injustices that may arise from minimal state intervention and a lack of redistributive policies. They argue that without government intervention, vulnerable populations may be left without adequate support or protection, leading to social disparities and injustices. Libertarian justice, championed by philosophers like Robert Nozick, emphasizes individual rights, freedoms, and limited state intervention. This theory rejects wealth redistribution, except in cases of rectifying past wrongs, and advocates for a minimal state focused on protecting individual rights and property. By prioritizing individual autonomy and voluntary interactions, libertarian justice offers a distinct perspective on justice and governance in society.

Egalitarian Justice:

Egalitarian theories of justice, like those proposed by John Rawls, emphasize equality in the distribution of goods and opportunities. Rawls' theory, for instance, includes the "difference principle," which allows for inequalities only if they benefit the least advantaged members of society. Egalitarian justice, as articulated in theories proposed by philosophers like John Rawls, underscores the importance of equality in the distribution of goods and opportunities within society. John Rawls, in his seminal work "A Theory of Justice," presents a framework for justice that prioritizes fairness and equal access to resources for all individuals.

Central to Rawls' theory of justice is the "difference principle," which permits inequalities in the distribution of goods and opportunities only if they result in benefits for the least advantaged members of society. This principle aims to address social and economic inequalities by ensuring that any disparities serve to improve the well-being of the most vulnerable individuals in society. Rawls argues that a just society is one where individuals have equal access to basic rights, liberties, and opportunities, regardless of their social or economic status. He proposes the concept of the "original position," where individuals make decisions about justice behind a "veil of ignorance" that obscures their own characteristics and circumstances. This thought experiment is designed to ensure impartiality and fairness in determining principles of justice that would be acceptable to all members of society. Egalitarian theories of justice, such as Rawls', advocate for redistributive policies and social programs aimed at reducing inequalities and promoting equal opportunities for all individuals. These theories challenge existing social structures and economic systems that perpetuate disparities and advocate for measures to uplift marginalized and disadvantaged groups.

Communitarian Justice:

Communitarianism, represented by philosophers like Michael Sandel, emphasizes the role of cultural norms and community values in shaping justice. It critiques liberal and libertarian models for overlooking the communal contexts that give meaning to individual choices. Communitarian justice, as advocated by philosophers like Michael Sandel, emphasizes the significance of cultural norms and community values in shaping notions of justice. This perspective critiques liberal and libertarian models for overlooking the communal contexts that give meaning to individual choices. Communitarianism underscores the importance of considering the impact of community values on ethical decision-making and societal well-being.

Michael Sandel, a prominent communitarian thinker, challenges the idea that justice can be divorced from communal values and argues that individual choices are deeply intertwined with the cultural and social contexts in which they occur. Sandel's work delves into the complexities of justice within communities and highlights the need to incorporate communal perspectives into ethical and political discourse. Communitarian justice stands in contrast to theories that prioritize individual autonomy and rights above communal values. It posits that justice cannot be fully understood or achieved without taking into account the shared norms, traditions, and values that shape communities.

By emphasizing the role of community in shaping ethical frameworks, communitarianism offers a nuanced perspective on justice that considers the broader social context in which decisions are made. In practical terms, communitarian justice calls for a reevaluation of how policies and practices impact communities and emphasizes the importance of fostering solidarity and mutual respect within society. This approach challenges the notion that justice can be solely based on individual rights and freedoms, advocating instead for a more holistic understanding of justice that incorporates communal well-being and values. Overall, communitarian justice offers a valuable perspective on ethical decision-making by highlighting the interconnectedness between individuals and their communities. By recognizing the influence of communal values on notions of justice, communitarianism enriches discussions on ethics and governance, promoting a more inclusive and culturally sensitive approach to justice in society.

Capability Approach:

Developed by Amartya Sen and further elaborated by Martha Nussbaum, this approach focuses on what individuals are able to do and be rather than merely what they have. It argues for a justice framework that ensures individuals have the freedom to achieve well-being, measured by capabilities rather than resources or utility. The Capability Approach, pioneered by Nobel laureate economist Amartya Sen and expanded upon by philosopher Martha Nussbaum, provides a unique perspective on justice that centers on individuals' capabilities and freedoms. This approach shifts the focus from traditional measures of well-being, such as income or resources, to what individuals are able to do and be.

The Capability Approach advocates for a justice framework that prioritizes enhancing individuals' capabilities to lead lives they value rather than solely focusing on material possessions or utility. Amartya Sen's seminal work on the Capability Approach challenges conventional economic theories that prioritize economic growth and material wealth as indicators of development. Sen argues that true development should be measured by individuals' capabilities to function effectively in society and pursue their own goals and aspirations. Central to Sen's approach is the concept of "capabilities," which refers to the real opportunities and freedoms that individuals have to lead lives they value.

Martha Nussbaum, a philosopher influenced by Sen's work, further expands on the Capability Approach by proposing a list of essential capabilities that are crucial for human flourishing. Nussbaum's capabilities include elements such as the ability to live a healthy life, to engage in meaningful relationships, to participate in political processes, and to have opportunities for personal development. By focusing on these fundamental capabilities, Nussbaum highlights the importance of enabling individuals to achieve a life of dignity and fulfillment. The Capability Approach offers a comprehensive framework for evaluating justice that goes beyond traditional measures of well-being, such as income or utility. Instead, it emphasizes the importance of expanding individuals' capabilities and freedoms to enable them to live lives that they have reason to value. The Capability Approach prioritizes human capabilities and agency, providing a more nuanced understanding of justice that considers the diverse needs and aspirations of individuals in society.

Procedural Justice:

This theory focuses on the fairness of the processes that lead to outcomes, rather than just the outcomes themselves. A just process is one that is consistent, unbiased, accurate, correctable, and representative of all affected interests. Procedural justice is a theory that emphasizes the fairness of the processes that lead to outcomes, rather than solely focusing on the outcomes themselves. This approach posits that a just process is characterized by several key principles, including consistency, impartiality, accuracy, correctability, and representation of all affected interests.

By prioritizing the fairness of procedures, procedural justice seeks to ensure that decision-making processes are transparent, equitable, and inclusive. Consistency is a fundamental aspect of procedural justice, requiring that similar cases be treated in a similar manner. This principle aims to promote predictability and uniformity in decision-making, reducing the likelihood of arbitrary or discriminatory outcomes. By adhering to consistent procedures, individuals can have confidence in the fairness and reliability of the system. Impartiality is another essential component of procedural justice, necessitating that decisions be made without bias or favoritism. An impartial process ensures that all individuals are treated fairly and without prejudice, regardless of their background, status, or characteristics.

By upholding impartiality, procedural justice seeks to safeguard the integrity and credibility of decision-making processes. Accuracy is a critical element of procedural justice, requiring that decisions be based on reliable information and evidence. An accurate process ensures that outcomes are informed by facts and data, rather than speculation or misinformation. By prioritizing accuracy, procedural justice aims to promote informed decision-making and minimize errors or inaccuracies that could lead to unjust outcomes. Correctability is a key principle of procedural justice that allows for errors or injustices to be rectified through mechanisms such as appeals or reviews. This principle acknowledges that no process is infallible and provides avenues for individuals to challenge decisions that they believe are unjust or incorrect. By incorporating correctability, procedural justice promotes accountability and transparency in decision-making processes. Representation of all affected interests is a crucial aspect of procedural justice, ensuring that the voices and perspectives of all stakeholders are considered in the decision-making process.

By including diverse viewpoints and ensuring that all affected parties have the opportunity to participate, procedural justice seeks to promote inclusivity and fairness in decision-making. Procedural justice is a theory that underscores the importance of fair processes in achieving just outcomes. By adhering to principles such as consistency, impartiality, accuracy, correctability, and representation of all affected interests, procedural justice aims to uphold fairness, transparency, and equity in decision-making processes. This approach emphasizes the importance of not only the decision results, but also the integrity and fairness of the procedures that lead to those outcomes.

Restorative Justice

Unlike retributive justice, which focuses on punishment, restorative justice seeks to heal and rebuild relationships by involving all stakeholders. This approach is often used in criminal justice systems to repair the harm caused by criminal behavior through cooperative processes that include all affected parties. Restorative justice is a paradigm that diverges from the traditional retributive justice model, which centers on punishment, by prioritizing the healing and restoration of relationships among all stakeholders involved. This approach is frequently employed in criminal justice systems to address the harm caused by criminal behavior through collaborative processes that engage all affected parties.

Restorative justice aims to repair the damage, promote accountability, and foster reconciliation by emphasizing dialogue, empathy, and active participation from those impacted by the wrongdoing. Restorative justice practices encompass a range of approaches, including victim-offender mediation, family group conferencing, and circle sentencing, among others. These processes provide opportunities for victims to express their needs and experiences, offenders to take responsibility for their actions, and communities to play a role in addressing the underlying causes of harm. By involving all stakeholders in a constructive and inclusive manner, restorative justice seeks to promote healing, understanding, and the rebuilding of relationships that have been fractured by criminal behavior.

Marxist Justice

Based on Karl Marx's ideas, this theory critiques capitalist systems and proposes that justice can only arise through the elimination of class structures and the distribution of resources according to need, not market dynamics. Marxist justice, rooted in Karl Marx's ideas, offers a critical perspective on capitalist systems and advocates for a radical restructuring of society to achieve justice by abolishing class distinctions and redistributing resources based on need rather than market forces.

This theory challenges the inherent inequalities and exploitative nature of capitalist economies, proposing a vision of justice that prioritizes the collective well-being of all individuals over profit-driven motives. Karl Marx, a prominent philosopher and economist, critiqued capitalism for perpetuating social divisions, alienating workers from the fruits of their labor, and concentrating wealth and power in the hands of a privileged few. Marxist justice contends that true justice can only be achieved by dismantling the capitalist system, which Marx viewed as inherently unjust due to its exploitation of labor and perpetuation of class disparities.

Central to Marxist justice is the concept of class struggle, which posits that society is divided into two conflicting classes – the bourgeoisie (capitalist class) and the proletariat (working class). Marx argued that the capitalist mode of production inherently generates inequality and alienation, as workers are exploited for profit by the owners of the means of production. In order to achieve justice, Marx proposed the abolition of private property, the means of production being owned collectively, and the establishment of a classless society where resources are distributed according to need.

Marxist justice challenges the notion that justice can be achieved through market mechanisms or individual accumulation of wealth. Instead, it advocates for a system where resources are allocated based on human needs, with the goal of ensuring equality, solidarity, and social harmony. By prioritizing the well-being of the collective over individual profit, Marxist justice seeks to create a society free from exploitation, oppression, and class-based inequalities.

Rawlsian Justice

John Rawls' principles, especially the difference principle, are relevant in ensuring that social and economic inequalities in healthcare are arranged so that they are to the greatest benefit of the least advantaged. This principle can guide policies on healthcare subsidies and support for vulnerable populations. Rawlsian justice, as articulated by the philosopher John Rawls, provides a framework for addressing social and economic inequalities in healthcare to benefit the least advantaged members of society. Central to Rawls' principles is the "difference principle," which asserts that inequalities should be structured in a way that maximizes the well-being of the most vulnerable individuals.

This principle can serve as a guiding force in shaping policies related to healthcare subsidies and support for marginalized populations. Rawlsian justice emphasizes the importance of ensuring that resources and services are distributed equitably in healthcare to address the needs of those who are least well-off. This principle challenges existing disparities in access to healthcare and advocates for policies that prioritize the health and well-being of vulnerable populations. Rawls' theory of justice has significant implications for healthcare policy development, particularly in areas such as healthcare subsidies, insurance coverage, and support for underserved communities. By applying the principles of Rawlsian justice, policymakers can design interventions that aim to reduce health inequalities, improve healthcare access, and enhance the quality of care for those who are most disadvantaged.

Communitarian Justice

Communitarian perspectives are valuable in contexts where community values and traditions have an impact on health practices and decisions. This approach can influence public health initiatives and policies that need to be culturally sensitive and community-oriented. Communitarian justice offers a valuable framework for addressing public health issues in contexts where community values and traditions play a significant role in shaping health practices and decisions. This approach emphasizes the importance of considering cultural context and community perspectives in designing public health initiatives and policies that are culturally sensitive and community-oriented. In the realm of public health, communitarian perspectives can inform strategies that prioritize community engagement, collaboration, and empowerment.

By recognizing the influence of community values on health behaviors and outcomes, public health interventions can be tailored to align with local norms and practices, thereby enhancing their effectiveness and acceptance within the community. One example of communitarian justice influencing public health initiatives is the promotion of culturally appropriate healthcare services for marginalized or underserved communities. By incorporating community values and traditions into healthcare delivery, providers can build trust, improve access to care, and address health disparities more effectively. Additionally, communitarian approaches can guide efforts to address public health challenges such as infectious diseases, chronic conditions, and mental health issues within diverse communities. By involving community members in the design and implementation of health programs, policymakers and practitioners can ensure that interventions are responsive to local needs and preferences, leading to better health outcomes and sustained behavior change.

CHAPTER KEY TERMS

Anarchy, State, and Utopia - A book by Robert Nozick that articulates the principles of libertarian justice, arguing for a minimal state focused solely on protecting individual rights, such as life, liberty, and property.

Capability Approach - A theory developed by Amartya Sen and Martha Nussbaum focusing on individuals' capabilities and freedoms, advocating for a justice framework that enhances individuals' ability to lead lives they value, beyond just having resources.

Communitarian Justice - A theory represented by philosophers like Michael Sandel, emphasizing the importance of cultural norms and community values in shaping justice. It critiques models that ignore communal contexts that give meaning to individual choices.

Difference Principle - Part of John Rawls' theory, which states that inequalities in social and economic arrangements are only just if they result in compensating benefits for the least advantaged members of society.

Egalitarian Justice - Theories, such as those proposed by John Rawls, that emphasize equality in the distribution of goods and opportunities, supporting the idea that benefits should favor the least advantaged in society.

Libertarian Justice - A theory advocated by Robert Nozick, focusing on the protection of individual rights and freedoms, and arguing against the redistribution of wealth except as compensation for past injustices.

Marxist Justice - Based on Karl Marx's critique of capitalist systems, this theory proposes that justice can be achieved only by eliminating class structures and redistributing resources according to need, not market dynamics.

Procedural Justice - A theory that emphasizes the fairness of processes that lead to outcomes, focusing on aspects like consistency, impartiality, accuracy, correctability, and the representation of all affected interests.

Restorative Justice - An approach that seeks to repair the harm caused by criminal behavior through cooperative processes involving all stakeholders, focusing on healing and rebuilding relationships rather than punitive measures.

Utilitarian Justice - Based on the principle of utilitarianism by philosophers like Jeremy Bentham, this theory advocates for actions that maximize overall happiness and minimize suffering, aiming for the greatest good for the greatest number.

DISCUSSION QUESTIONS

1. **Utilitarian Justice**: Imagine a government has to decide between two health policies: one that benefits a small group of seriously ill patients or another that moderately improves the health of a

much larger population. How would a utilitarian justify choosing one policy over the other?

2. **Capability Approach**: Consider a scenario where a rural community lacks access to higher education. How might the Capability Approach argue for interventions in this community, and what specific capabilities might it aim to enhance?

3. **Libertarian Justice**: In a town experiencing rapid industrial growth, residents are suffering from increased pollution. The government wants to impose strict environmental regulations on the factories. How would a proponent of libertarian justice view these regulations?

4. **Rawlsian Justice**: Imagine a society where a new policy is proposed that will increase taxes on the wealthy to fund better public transportation, which primarily benefits the less affluent. How would the difference principle apply to this policy?

5. **Communitarian Justice**: A new law requires that individuals from different cultural backgrounds must perform community service together to promote social cohesion. How might a communitarian assess the potential benefits and drawbacks of this law?

6. **Restorative Justice**: Suppose a juvenile delinquent is caught vandalizing public property. Instead of traditional punishment, the court considers a restorative justice approach. What process might be involved, and how could it benefit both the community and the offender?

7. **Marxist Justice**: Imagine a country where the wealth generated by automation is owned by a small group of capitalists, while a large portion of the population remains unemployed. How would a Marxist theorist propose restructuring this society?

8. **Procedural Justice**: A company is caught discriminating against certain applicants during its hiring process. What steps should

be taken to ensure procedural justice in revising the company's hiring practices?

9. **Capability Approach:** In a developing country, a foreign aid program aims to improve living conditions. Should the program focus more on providing resources like food and water, or enhancing capabilities such as education and healthcare? Why might Amartya Sen advocate for one approach over the other?

10. **Libertarian Justice:** Suppose a government considers making vaccination mandatory to combat a public health crisis. How might a libertarian argue for or against this mandate based on individual rights and freedoms?

REFERENCES

Albanesi, B., Marchetti, A., D'Angelo, D., Capuzzo, M., Mastroianni, C., Artico, M., ... & Marinis, M. (2020). Exploring nurses' involvement in artificial nutrition and hydration at the end of life: a scoping review. Journal of Parenteral and Enteral Nutrition, 44(7), 1220-1233. https://doi.org/10.1002/jpen.1772

Amann, J., Blasimme, A., Frey, D., & Madai, V. (2020). Explainability for artificial intelligence in healthcare: a multidisciplinary perspective. BMC Medical Informatics and Decision Making, 20(1). https://doi.org/10.1186/s12911-020-01332-6

Ando, S., Yamaguchi, S., Aoki, Y., & Thornicroft, G. (2013). Review of mental-health-related stigma in japan. Psychiatry and Clinical Neurosciences, 67(7), 471-482. https://doi.org/10.1111/pcn.12086

Arciniegas, D. (2015). Psychosis. Continuum Lifelong Learning in Neurology, 21, 715-736. https://doi.org/10.1212/01.con.0000466662.89908.e7

Arlinghaus, R., Schwab, A., Cooke, S., & Cowx, I. (2009). Contrasting pragmatic and suffering-centred approaches to fish welfare in recreational angling. Journal of Fish

Armstrong, A. (2006). Towards a strong virtue ethics for nursing practice. Nursing Philosophy, 7(3), 110-124. https://doi.org/10.1111/j.1466-769x.2006.00268.x

Aten, J., Topping, S., Denney, R., & Bayne, T. (2010). Collaborating with african american churches to overcome minority disaster mental health disparities: what mental health professionals can learn from hurricane katrina.. Professional Psychology Research and Practice, 41(2), 167-173. https://doi.org/10.1037/a0018116

Baeke, G., Wils, J., & Broeckaert, B. (2011). 'there is a time to be born and a time to die' (ecclesiastes 3:2a): jewish perspectives on euthanasia. Journal of Religion and Health, 50(4), 778-795. https://doi.org/10.1007/s10943-011-9465-9

Baertschi, B. (2014). Human dignity as a component of a long-lasting and widespread conceptual construct. Journal of Bioethical Inquiry, 11(2), 201-211. https://doi.org/10.1007/s11673-014-9512-9

Balzer, M., Clajus, C., Eden, G., Euteneuer, F., Haller, H., Martin, H., ... & Fuerholzer, K. (2019). Patient perspectives on renal replacement therapy modality choice: a multicenter questionnaire study on bioethical dimensions. Peritoneal Dialysis International, 39(6), 519-526. https://doi.org/10.3747/pdi.2018.00285

Baradaran, H., Gorgzadeh, N., Seraj, H., Asadi, A., Shamshirian, D., & Rezapour, M. (2020). Drug-drug interaction between psychiatric medications and experimental treatments for coronavirus disease-19: a mini-review. Open Access Macedonian Journal of Medical Sciences, 8(T1), 216-228. https://doi.org/10.3889/oamjms.2020.5010

Becker, S. and Forman, H. (2020). Implied consent in treating psychiatric emergencies. Frontiers in Psychiatry, 11. https://doi.org/10.3389/fpsyt.2020.00127

Benatar, S. (2003). Public health and public health ethics. Acta Bioethica, 9(2). https://doi.org/10.4067/s1726-569x2003000200006

Benatar, S. and Upshur, R. (2014). Virtues and values in medicine revisited: individual and global health. Clinical Medicine, 14(5), 495-499. https://doi.org/10.7861/clinmedicine.14-5-495

Berlan, E. and Bravender, T. (2009). Confidentiality, consent, and caring for the adolescent patient. Current Opinion in Pediatrics, 21(4), 450-456. https://doi.org/10.1097/mop.0b013e32832ce009

Blomqvist, H., Bergdahl, E., & Hemberg, J. (2022). Ethical sensitivity and compassion in home care: leaders' views. Nursing Ethics, 30(2), 180-196. https://doi.org/10.1177/09697330221122965

Borgstrom, E. and Walter, T. (2015). Choice and compassion at the end of life: a critical analysis of recent english policy discourse. Social Science & Medicine, 136-137, 99-105. https://doi.org/10.1016/j.socscimed.2015.05.013

Boylan, M. (2016). Ethical dimensions of mathematics education. Educational Studies in Mathematics, 92(3), 395-409. https://doi.org/10.1007/s10649-015-9678-z

Butchart, L. (2022). Taoism, bioethics, and the covid-19 pandemic. Tzu Chi Medical Journal, 34(1), 107. https://doi.org/10.4103/tcmj.tcmj_77_21

Catts, O. and Zurr, I. (2018). Artists working with life (sciences) in contestable settings. Interdisciplinary Science Reviews, 43(1), 40-53. https://doi.org/10.1080/03080188.2018.1418122

Cajiao, X. (2023). Colombia and medical tourism. Voices in Bioethics, 9. https://doi.org/10.52214/vib.v9i.11941

Carson, T. (2013). Golden rule.. https://doi.org/10.1002/9781444367072.wbiee188Kinnier, R., Kernes, J., & Dautheribes, T. (2000). A short list of universal moral values. Counseling and Values, 45(1), 4-16. https://doi.org/10.1002/j.2161-007x.2000.tb00178.x

Chervenak, F. and McCullough, L. (2017). Ethical dimensions of the fetus as a patient. Best Practice & Research Clinical Obstetrics & Gynaecology, 43, 2-9. https://doi.org/10.1016/j. bpobgyn.2016.12.007

Chukwuneke, F., Umeora, O., Maduabuchi, J., & Egbunike, N. (2014). Global bioethics and culture in a pluralistic world: how does culture influence bioethics in africa?. Annals of Medical and Health Sciences Research, 4(5), 672. https://doi. org/10.4103/2141-9248.141495

Clausen, L., Larsen, J., Bulik, C., & Petersen, L. (2018). A danish register-based study on involuntary treatment in anorexia nervosa. International Journal of Eating Disorders, 51(11), 1213-1222. https://doi.org/10.1002/eat.22968

Cohen, J., Delden, J., Mortier, F., Löfmark, R., Norup, M., Cartwright, C., ... & Bilsen, J. (2008). Influence of physicians' life stances on attitudes to end-of-life decisions and actual end-of-life decision-making in six countries. Journal of Medical Ethics, 34(4), 247-253. https://doi.org/10.1136/jme.2006.020297

Conrad, R., Baum, M., Shah, S., Levy-Carrick, N., Biswas, J., Schmelzer, N., ... & Silbersweig, D. (2020). Duties toward patients with psychiatric illness. The Hastings Center Report, 50(3), 67-69. https://doi.org/10.1002/hast.1139

Cooper, D. (2021). The case for compulsory surgical smoke evacuation systems in the operating theatre. Clinical Ethics, 17(2), 130-135. https://doi.org/10.1177/14777509211063589

Couture, V., Dubois, M., Drouin, R., Moutquin, J., & Bouffard, C. (2014). Strengths and pitfalls of canadian gamete and embryo donor registries: searching for beneficent solutions. Reproductive Biomedicine Online, 28(3), 369-379. https://doi.org/10.1016/j. rbmo.2013.10.020

Dahl, A. (2023). What we do when we define morality (and why we need to do it).. https://doi.org/10.31219/osf.io/uvkw4

Dangi, T. and Petrick, J. (2021). Augmenting the role of tourism governance in addressing destination justice, ethics, and equity for sustainable community-based tourism. Tourism and Hospitality, 2(1), 15-42. https://doi.org/10.3390/tourhosp2010002

Djamaluddin, N., Anwar, A., Sadad, R., R.A.P, F., & Wulansari, D. (2019). The effect of duration of antipsychotics medicine use toward the salivary flow rate of schizophrenics in special hospital of south sulawesi province.. https://doi.org/10.4108/eai.26-10-2018.2288940

Dobrin, M., Voinea, A., Rădulescu, I., & Nechita, P. (2019). Involuntary psychiatric admission – a comparison between legal frameworks. Bulletin of Integrative Psychiatry, 25(3), 66-74. https://doi.org/10.36219/bpi.2019.03.06

Doukas, D. (2003). Where is the virtue in professionalism?. Cambridge Quarterly of Healthcare Ethics, 12(2), 147-154. https://doi.org/10.1017/s0963180103122037

Drezgić, R. (2012). On feminist engagements with bioethics. Filozofija I Drustvo, 23(4), 19-31. https://doi.org/10.2298/fid1204019d

English, D. (2005). Moral obligations of patients: a clinical view. The Journal of Medicine and Philosophy a Forum for Bioethics and Philosophy of Medicine, 30(2), 139-152. https://doi.org/10.1080/03605310590926821

Ergin, A., Özcan, M., & Aksoy, S. (2019). The compassion levels of midwives working in the delivery room. Nursing Ethics, 27(3), 887-898. https://doi.org/10.1177/0969733019874495

Fairchild, A. (2020). The role of compassion in ethical frameworks and medical practice. Clinical Ethics, 16(4), 302-306. https://doi.org/10.1177/1477750920983572

Forouzan, S., Padyab, M., Rafiey, H., Ghazinour, M., Dejman, M., & Sebastian, M. (2016). Measuring the mental health-care system responsiveness: results of an outpatient survey in tehran. Frontiers in Public Health, 3. https://doi.org/10.3389/fpubh.2015.00285

Galdames, I., Fuentes, M., Jurado, M., Martínez, Á., Márquez, M., Martín, A., ... & Linares, J. (2020). Moral sensitivity, empathy and prosocial behavior: implications for humanization of nursing care. International Journal of Environmental Research and Public Health, 17(23), 8914. https://doi.org/10.3390/ijerph17238914

Giblin, M. (1997). The prophetic role of feminist bioethics. Horizons, 24(1), 37-49. https://doi.org/10.1017/s0360966900016728

Gielen, J., Branden, S., & Broeckaert, B. (2009). Religion and nurses' attitudes to euthanasia and physician assisted suicide. Nursing Ethics, 16(3), 303-318. https://doi.org/10.1177/0969733009102692

Glick, S. (2012). Synthetic biology: a jewish view. Perspectives in Biology and Medicine, 55(4), 571-580. https://doi.org/10.1353/pbm.2012.0039

Goodpaster, K. (2017). Human dignity and the common good: the institutional insight. Business and Society Review, 122(1), 27-50. https://doi.org/10.1111/basr.12107

Greenfield, B. and West, C. (2012). Ethical issues in sports medicine. Sports Health a Multidisciplinary Approach, 4(6), 475-479. https://doi.org/10.1177/1941738112459327

Häyry, M. (2020). Just better utilitarianism. Cambridge Quarterly of Healthcare Ethics, 30(2), 343-367. https://doi.org/10.1017/s0963180120000882

Hedgecoe, A. (2009). Bioethics and the reinforcement of socio-technical expectations. Social Studies of Science, 40(2), 163-186. https://doi.org/10.1177/0306312709349781

Hem, M., Molewijk, B., & Pedersen, R. (2014). Ethical challenges in connection with the use of coercion: a focus group study of health care personnel in mental health care. BMC Medical Ethics, 15(1). https://doi.org/10.1186/1472-6939-15-82

Hem, M., Gjerberg, E., Husum, T., & Pedersen, R. (2016). Ethical challenges when using coercion in mental healthcare: a systematic literature review. Nursing Ethics, 25(1), 92-110. https://doi.org/10.1177/0969733016629770

Herissone-Kelly, P. (2022). How to deal with counter-examples to common morality theory: a surprising result. Cambridge Quarterly of Healthcare Ethics, 31(2), 185-191. https://doi.org/10.1017/s096318012100058x

Herreros, B., Benito, M., Gella, P., Valenti, E., Sánchez, B., & Velasco, T. (2020). Why have advance directives failed in spain?. BMC Medical Ethics, 21(1). https://doi.org/10.1186/s12910-020-00557-4

Hodgson, J., Mendenhall, T., & Lamson, A. (2013). Patient and provider relationships: consent, confidentiality, and managing mistakes in integrated primary care settings.. Families Systems & Health, 31(1), 28-40. https://doi.org/10.1037/a0031771

Hofstad, T., Husum, T., Rugkåsa, J., & Hofmann, B. (2022). Geographical variation in compulsory hospitalisation – ethical challenges. BMC Health Services Research, 22(1). https://doi.org/10.1186/s12913-022-08798-2

Hunt, M. and Godard, B. (2013). Beyond procedural ethics: foregrounding questions of justice in global health research ethics training for students. Global Public Health, 8(6), 713-724. https://doi.org/10.1080/17441692.2013.796400

Ilesanmi, S. (2023). Religious ethics and the human dignity revolution. Journal of Religious Ethics, 51(4), 652-672. https://doi.org/10.1111/jore.12465

Iltis, A. (2018). Engelhardt on the common morality in bioethics. Conatus, 3(2), 49. https://doi.org/10.12681/conatus.19284

Jameson, M. and Naugle, A. (2013). Attitudes toward empirically-supported treatments among pastoral mental health care providers: exploratory findings and future directions. Journal of Pastoral Care & Counseling Advancing Theory and Professional Practice Through Scholarly and Reflective Publications, 67(3), 1-12. https://doi.org/10.1177/154230501306700305

Jo, H. and Kim, S. (2017). Moral sensitivity, empathy and perceived ethical climate of psychiatric nurses working in the national mental hospitals. Journal of Korean Academy of Psychiatric and Mental Health Nursing, 26(2), 204. https://doi.org/10.12934/jkpmhn.2017.26.2.204

Joury, S., Asman, O., & Gold, A. (2023). Caregivers' perceptions of compulsory treatment of physical illness in involuntarily psychiatric hospitalization. Nursing Ethics, 30(3), 423-436. https://doi.org/10.1177/09697330221140493

Joury, S., Asman, O., & Gold, A. (2023). Caregivers' perceptions of compulsory treatment of physical illness in involuntarily psychiatric hospitalization. Nursing Ethics, 30(3), 423-436. https://doi.org/10.1177/09697330221140493

Kane, M., Green, D., & Jacobs, R. (2011). Pastoral care professionals in health and mental health care: recognizing classic and newer versions of ageism. Journal of Pastoral Care & Counseling Advancing Theory and Professional Practice Through Scholarly and Reflective Publications, 65(4), 1-9. https://doi.org/10.1177/154230501106500405

Kanner, A. (2016). Management of psychiatric and neurological comorbidities in epilepsy. Nature Reviews Neurology, 12(2), 106-116. https://doi.org/10.1038/nrneurol.2015.243

Kavussanu, M. and Al-Yaaribi, A. (2019). Prosocial and antisocial behaviour in sport. International Journal of Sport and Exercise Psychology, 19(2), 179-202. https://doi.org/10.1080/1612197x.2019.1674681

Koslander, T., Silva, A., & Roxberg, Å. (2009). Existential and spiritual needs in mental health care. Journal of Holistic Nursing, 27(1), 34-42. https://doi.org/10.1177/0898010108323302

Kullgren, G., Jacobsson, L., Lynøe, N., Kohn, R., & Levav, I. (1996). Practices and attitudes among swedish psychiatrists regarding the ethics of compulsory treatment. Acta Psychiatrica Scandinavica, 93(5), 389-396. https://doi.org/10.1111/j.1600-0447.1996.tb10665.x

Kvaran, T. and Sanfey, A. (2010). Toward an integrated neuroscience of morality: the contribution of neuroeconomics to moral cognition. Topics in Cognitive Science, 2(3), 579-595. https://doi.org/10.1111/j.1756-8765.2010.01086.x

Laakasuo, M., Palomäki, J., Kunnari, A., Rauhala, S., Drosinou, M., Halonen, J., … & Francis, K. (2022). Moral psychology of nursing robots: exploring the role of robots in dilemmas of patient autonomy. European Journal of Social Psychology, 53(1), 108-128. https://doi.org/10.1002/ejsp.2890

Lebacqz, K. (2016). On hope and hard choices. Journal of Religious Ethics, 44(4), 722-737. https://doi.org/10.1111/jore.12157

Lertxundi, U., Domingo-Echaburu, S., Hernández, R., Peral, J., & Medrano, J. (2013). Expert-based drug lists to measure anticholinergic burden: similar names, different results. Psychogeriatrics, 13(1), 17-24. https://doi.org/10.1111/j.1479-8301.2012.00418.x

Lester, H., Miwa, J., & Srinivasan, R. (2012). Psychiatric drugs bind to classical targets within early exocytotic pathways: therapeutic effects. Biological Psychiatry, 72(11), 907-915. https://doi.org/10.1016/j.biopsych.2012.05.020

Li, J., He, D., Zhang, W., Huang, R., & He, X. (2023). The effect of moral behavior on facial attractiveness. Psychology Research and Behavior Management, Volume 16, 1521-1532. https://doi.org/10.2147/prbm.s408741

Lustgarten, S., Garrison, Y., Sinnard, M., & Flynn, A. (2020). Digital privacy in mental healthcare: current issues and recommendations for technology use. Current Opinion in Psychology, 36, 25-31. https://doi.org/10.1016/j.copsyc.2020.03.012

Madadin, M., Sahwan, H., Altarouti, K., Altarouti, S., Eswaikt, Z., & Menezes, R. (2020). The islamic perspective on physician-assisted suicide and euthanasia. Medicine Science and the Law, 60(4), 278-286. https://doi.org/10.1177/0025802420934241

Magelssen, M., Holmøy, T., Horn, M., Dybwik, K., & Førde, R. (2018). Ethical challenges in tracheostomy-assisted ventilation in amyotrophic lateral sclerosis. Journal of Neurology, 265(11), 2730-2736. https://doi.org/10.1007/s00415-018-9054-x

Mammì, A., Ferlazzo, E., Gasparini, S., Bova, V., Neri, S., Labate, A., ... & Aguglia, U. (2022). Psychiatric and behavioural side effects associated with perampanel in patients with temporal lobe epilepsy.

a real-world experience. Frontiers in Neurology, 13. https://doi. org/10.3389/fneur.2022.839985

Martinho, S., Santa-Rosa, B., & Silvestre, M. (2022). Where the public health principles meet the individual: a framework for the ethics of compulsory outpatient treatment in psychiatry. BMC Medical Ethics, 23(1). https://doi.org/10.1186/s12910-022-00814-8

Mathieu, R. (2016). Jewish ethics and xenotransplantation. Xenotransplantation, 23(4), 258-268. https://doi.org/10.1111/xen.12247

McGlothen-Bell, K., McGrath, J., Brownell, E., Shlafer, R., & Crawford, A. (2022). Applying a reproductive justice lens to enhance research engagement among systematically underrepresented childbearing women. Nursing Research, 72(2), 132-140. https:// doi.org/10.1097/nnr.0000000000000639

Molewijk, B., Engerdahl, I., & Pedersen, R. (2016). Two years of moral case deliberations on the use of coercion in mental health care: which ethical challenges are being discussed by health care professionals?. Clinical Ethics, 11(2-3), 87-96. https://doi. org/10.1177/1477750915622034

Morales-Sánchez, R. and Cabello-Medina, C. (2015). Integrating character in management: virtues, character strengths, and competencies. Business Ethics a European Review, 24(S2). https://doi. org/10.1111/beer.12104

Moynihan, K., Dorste, A., Siegel, B., Rabinowitz, E., McReynolds, A., & October, T. (2021). Decision-making, ethics, and end-of-life care in pediatric extracorporeal membrane oxygenation: a comprehensive narrative review. Pediatric Critical Care Medicine, 22(9), 806-812. https://doi.org/10.1097/pcc.0000000000002766

Naphan-Kingery, D., Miles, M., Brockman, A., McKane, R., Botchway, P., & McGee, E. (2019). Investigation of an equity ethic in engineering and computing doctoral students. Journal of Engineering Education, 108(3), 337-354. https://doi.org/10.1002/jee.20284

Ndumbe-Eyoh, S., Muzumdar, P., Betker, C., & Oickle, D. (2021).'back to better': amplifying health equity, and determinants of health perspectives during the covid-19 pandemic. Global Health Promotion, 28(2), 7-16. https://doi.org/10.1177/17579759211000975

Nechita, P., Luca, L., Voinea, A., Moraru, C., & Dobri, M. (2020). Coercive measures and stigmatization in the psychiatric medical care. Brain Broad Research in Artificial Intelligence and Neuroscience, 11(3sup1), 137-145. https://doi.org/10.18662/brain/11.3sup1/129

Nieuwsma, J., Fortune-Greeley, A., Jackson, G., Meador, K., Beckham, J., & Elbogen, E. (2014). Pastoral care use among post-9/11 veterans who screen positive for mental health problems.. Psychological Services, 11(3), 300-308. https://doi.org/10.1037/a0037065

Norvoll, R., Hem, M., & Pedersen, R. (2016). The role of ethics in reducing and improving the quality of coercion in mental health care. Hec Forum, 29(1), 59-74. https://doi.org/10.1007/s10730-016-9312-1

Oakley, J. and Cocking, D. (2001). Virtue ethics and professional roles.. https://doi.org/10.1017/cbo9780511487118

O'Brien, A. and Golding, C. (2003). Coercion in mental healthcare: the principle of least coercive care. Journal of Psychiatric and Mental Health Nursing, 10(2), 167-173. https://doi.org/10.1046/j.1365-2850.2003.00571.x

Okoro, R. and Biambo, A. (2020). Pharmacy students' perceived professionalism and application of bioethical principles: implications for teaching pharmacy ethics for patient-centred pharmacy practice. Pharmacy Education, 20, 158-167. https://doi.org/10.46542/pe.2020.201.158167

Ortega-Galán, Á., Pérez-García, E., Brito-Pons, G., Ramos-Pichardo, J., Carmona-Rega, M., & Fernández, M. (2021). Understanding the concept of compassion from the perspectives of nurses. Nursing Ethics, 28(6), 996-1009. https://doi.org/10.1177/0969733020983401

P, Deepa. (2020). Individual dignity and euthanasia: an ethical perspective. Global Bioethics Enquiry Journal, 8(1), 46. https://doi.org/10.38020/gbe.8.1.2020.46-49

Padela, A. and Mohiuddin, A. (2015). Ethical obligations and clinical goals in end-of-life care: deriving a quality-of-life construct based on the islamic concept of accountability before god (taklīf). The American Journal of Bioethics, 15(1), 3-13. https://doi.org/10.1080/15265161.2014.974769

Poel, I. (2015). An ethical framework for evaluating experimental technology. Science and Engineering Ethics, 22(3), 667-686. https://doi.org/10.1007/s11948-015-9724-3

Purificacion, S., French, J., & d'Agincourt-Canning, L. (2015). Inequities in access to cancer care in canada. Healthcare Management Forum, 28(6), 265-269. https://doi.org/10.1177/0840470415599136

Quaghebeur, T., Casterlé, B., & Gastmans, C. (2009). Nursing and euthanasia: a review of argument-based ethics literature. Nursing Ethics, 16(4), 466-486. https://doi.org/10.1177/0969733009104610

Rezapour-Mirsaleh, Y., Aghabagheri, M., Choobforoushzadeh, A., & Ardakan, A. (2021). Mindfulness, empathy and moral sensitivity

in nurses: a structural equation modeling analysis.. https://doi.
org/10.21203/rs.3.rs-821194/v1

Richards, D., Khan, S., Formosa, P., & Bankins, S. (2022). The influence
of ethical principles and policy awareness priming on university students' judgements about ict code of conduct compliance.
Organizational Cybersecurity Journal Practice Process and People, 2(2), 134-161. https://doi.org/10.1108/ocj-01-2022-0001

Richardson, S. and Weaver, K. (2016). Vaccinate-or-mask: ethical duties
and rights of health care providers in obtaining or refusing the
influenza vaccination. Clinical Ethics, 11(4), 182-189. https://
doi.org/10.1177/1477750916657663

Robertson, M., Ryan, C., & Walter, G. (2007). Overview of psychiatric
ethics iv: the method of casuistry. Australasian Psychiatry, 15(4),
287-291. https://doi.org/10.1080/10398560701378582

Robins–Browne, K., Guillemin, M., Hegarty, K., & Palmer, V. (2018).
Bringing together the listening guide and moral self-definition
for narrative analysis of older people's understanding of health-
related decision-making. Qualitative Research, 19(5), 594-610.
https://doi.org/10.1177/1468794118786613

Robson, A. (2022). Aquinas's principle of misericordia in corporations:
implications for workers and other stakeholders. Humanistic
Management Journal, 7(2), 233-257. https://doi.org/10.1007/
s41463-022-00137-1

Rueda, J. (2022). Genetic enhancement, human extinction, and the best
interests of posthumaniy. Bioethics. https://doi.org/10.1111/
bioe.13085

Rüsch, N., Müller, M., Lay, B., Corrigan, P., Zahn, R., Schönenberger,
T., ... & Rössler, W. (2013). Emotional reactions to involuntary psychiatric hospitalization and stigma-related stress among

people with mental illness. European Archives of Psychiatry and Clinical Neuroscience, 264(1), 35-43. https://doi.org/10.1007/s00406-013-0412-5

Santamaría-García, H., Báez, S., García, A., Flichtentrei, D., Prats, M., Mastandueno, R., ... & Ibáñez, A. (2017). Empathy for others' suffering and its mediators in mental health professionals. Scientific Reports, 7(1). https://doi.org/10.1038/s41598-017-06775-y

Sartwelle, T., Johnston, J., & Arda, B. (2015). Perpetuating myths, fables, and fairy tales: a half century of electronic fetal monitoring. The Surgery Journal, 01(01), e28-e34. https://doi.org/10.1055/s-0035-1567880

Savulescu, J. and Birks, D. (2012). Bioethics: utilitarianism. https://doi.org/10.1002/9780470015902.a0005891.pub2

Schenker, J. (2005). Assisted reproduction practice: religious perspectives. Reproductive Biomedicine Online, 10(3), 310-319. https://doi.org/10.1016/s1472-6483(10)61789-0

Shaffer, F., Álvarez, T., & Stievano, A. (2022). Guaranteeing dignity and decent work for migrant nurses and health care workers beyond the covid-19 pandemic. Journal of Nursing Management, 30(8), 3918-3921. https://doi.org/10.1111/jonm.13751

Shafiekhani, M. and Mirjalili, M. (2018). Psychotropic drug therapy in patients in the intensive care unit - usage, adverse effects and drug interactions: a review. Therapeutics and Clinical Risk Management, Volume 14, 1799-1812. https://doi.org/10.2147/tcrm.s176079

Shahzad, K., Murad, H., Kitchlew, N., & Zia, S. (2014). Integrating principles of care, compassion and justice in organizations: exploring dynamic nature of organizational justice. Journal of Human Values, 20(2), 167-181. https://doi.org/10.1177/0971685814539411

Shen, N., Sequeira, L., Silver, M., Carter-Langford, A., Strauss, J., & Wiljer, D. (2019). Patient privacy perspectives on health information exchange in a mental health context: qualitative study. Jmir Mental Health, 6(11), e13306. https://doi.org/10.2196/13306

Sjöstrand, M., Sandman, L., Karlsson, P., Helgesson, G., Eriksson, S., & Juth, N. (2015). Ethical deliberations about involuntary treatment: interviews with swedish psychiatrists. BMC Medical Ethics, 16(1). https://doi.org/10.1186/s12910-015-0029-5

Skogen, J., Sivertsen, B., Lundervold, A., Stormark, K., Jakobsen, R., & Hysing, M. (2014). Alcohol and drug use among adolescents: and the co-occurrence of mental health problems. ung@hordaland, a population-based study. BMJ Open, 4(9), e005357-e005357. https://doi.org/10.1136/bmjopen-2014-005357

Slater, M. and Banakou, D. (2021). The golden rule as a paradigm for fostering prosocial behavior with virtual reality. Current Directions in Psychological Science, 30(6), 503-509. https://doi.org/10.1177/09637214211046954

Starfield, B., Shi, L., & Macinko, J. (2005). Contribution of primary care to health systems and health. Milbank Quarterly, 83(3), 457-502. https://doi.org/10.1111/j.1468-0009.2005.00409.x

Smith, M., Thompson, A., & Upshur, R. (2018). Is 'health equity' bad for our health? a qualitative empirical ethics study of public health policy-makers' perspectives. Can J Public Health, 109(5-6), 633-642. https://doi.org/10.17269/s41997-018-0128-4

Smith-MacDonald, L., Venturato, L., Hunter, P., Kaasalainen, S., Sussman, T., McCleary, L., … & Sinclair, S. (2019). Perspectives and experiences of compassion in long-term care facilities within canada: a qualitative study of patients, family members and health care providers. BMC Geriatrics, 19(1). https://doi.org/10.1186/s12877-019-1135-x

Stievano, A., Mynttinen, M., Rocco, G., & Kangasniemi, M. (2022). Public health nurses' professional dignity: an interview study in finland. Nursing Ethics, 29(6), 1503-1517. https://doi.org/10.1177/09697330221107143

Susewind, M. and Hoelzl, E. (2014). A matter of perspective: why past moral behavior can sometimes encourage and other times discourage future moral striving. Journal of Applied Social Psychology, 44(3), 201-209. https://doi.org/10.1111/jasp.12214

Tarabeih, M. (2023). The view of the three monotheistic religions toward xenotransplantation. Clinical Transplantation, 38(1). https://doi.org/10.1111/ctr.15192

Tarsitani, L., Rocca, B., Pancheri, C., Biondi, M., Pasquini, M., Ferracuti, S., … & Mandarelli, G. (2021). Involuntary psychiatric hospitalization among migrants in italy: a matched sample study. International Journal of Social Psychiatry, 68(2), 429-434. https://doi.org/10.1177/00207640211001903

Tate, T. and Clair, J. (2023). Love your patient as yourself: on reviving the broken heart of american medical ethics. The Hastings Center Report, 53(2), 12-25. https://doi.org/10.1002/hast.1470

Valenti, E., Giacco, D., Katasakou, C., & Priebe, S. (2013). Which values are important for patients during involuntary treatment? a qualitative study with psychiatric inpatients. Journal of Medical Ethics, 40(12), 832-836. https://doi.org/10.1136/medethics-2011-100370

Varkey, B. (2020). Principles of clinical ethics and their application to practice. Medical Principles and Practice, 30(1), 17-28. https://doi.org/10.1159/000509119

Vuckovich, P. (2010). Compliance versus adherence in serious and persistent mental illness. Nursing Ethics, 17(1), 77-85. https://doi.org/10.1177/0969733009352047

Wahlert, L. and Fiester, A. (2011). Queer bioethics: why its time has come. Bioethics, 26(1). https://doi.org/10.1111/j.1467-8519.2011.01957.x

Wahlert, L. and Fiester, A. (2014). Repaving the road of good intentions: lgbt health care and the queer bioethical lens. The Hastings Center Report, 44(s4). https://doi.org/10.1002/hast.373

Wasserman, D., Apter, G., Baeken, C., Bailey, S., Balazs, J., Bec, C., ... & Vahip, S. (2020). Compulsory admissions of patients with mental disorders: state of the art on ethical and legislative aspects in 40 european countries. European Psychiatry, 63(1). https://doi.org/10.1192/j.eurpsy.2020.79

Wimberly, J. (2019). Virtue ethics and the commitment to learn: overcoming disparities faced by transgender individuals. Philosophy Ethics and Humanities in Medicine, 14(1). https://doi.org/10.1186/s13010-019-0079-2

Wynn, R. (2006). Coercion in psychiatric care: clinical, legal, and ethical controversies. International Journal of Psychiatry in Clinical Practice, 10(4), 247-251. https://doi.org/10.1080/13651500600650026

Yüksel, Ö., Günüşen, N., Ince, S., & Zeybekçi, S. (2022). Experiences of oncology nurses regarding self-compassion and compassionate care: a qualitative study. International Nursing Review, 69(4), 432-441. https://doi.org/10.1111/inr.12747

Zölzer, F. (2016). Are the core values of the radiological protection system shared across cultures?. Annals of the Icrp, 45(1_suppl), 358-372. https://doi.org/10.1177/0146645316630169

AUTHOR BIOGRAPHY

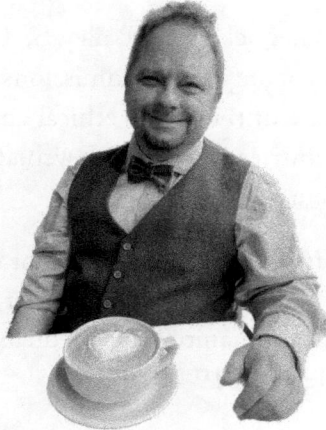

D r Rodgir Cohen is a university lecturer, educator, and community figure who brings a wealth of experience and insight into his teachings on bioethics and religion. At Loma Linda University, Rodgir delves into the complex intersections of bioethical issues with religious perspectives, engaging his students with thoughtful discourse and deep ethical considerations. Rodgir also lectures at California State University-Fullerton on a broad range of topics, including religions of the world, politics and religion, and psychology, and religion.

Having served in the armed forces during a significant time of conflict, he has firsthand experience of the harsh realities of war, which he leverages to enrich his teachings and activism. His transition from military life to academia and community service speaks volumes of his dedication and resilience. A family man at heart, he cherishes quality time with his loved ones. His interest in boating also offers him a peaceful retreat from his active professional life, allowing him moments of tranquility amidst nature.

www.ingramcontent.com/pod-product-compliance
Lightning Source LLC
Chambersburg PA
CBHW031940190326
41519CB00007B/591